"To articulate biblical sexual ethics in a secular society, two things are needed: first, a fierce loyalty to the author of those ethics, and second, an empathetic understanding of what it takes for people to come under that author's authority. This description reminds me of the Roman centurion who came to Jesus pleading on behalf of his sick servant. He cared about his servant. He had a pastor's heart. But he was a soldier and sensed the need to take this matter higher up the chain of command. He knew Jesus's rank and acknowledged his own unworthiness. He would honor whatever decision Jesus made, but he appealed to the Lord's grace. The centurion knew that only Jesus had the answer for his servant's sickness.

Jeff Schlenz is also a pastor and soldier, and because he is both, I trust him to handle the sensitive subject of sexual ethics. As a pastor, he sees the sexual confusion and sickness around him and longs for people to be healed. As a soldier, his instinct is to take this issue higher up the chain of command. He bows to the Savior, the true author of sexual ethics, and appeals to Jesus's willingness to help. Rev. Colonel Schlenz is just the person to uncover our confusion and bring us back to the healing of God's Word."

—Sandy Adams, pastor at Calvary Chapel Stone Mountain in Lilburn, GA

"As a counselor, I found this book both theologically rich and practically insightful. Written by a pastor who takes his calling seriously, it offers a clear and compassionate look at the brokenness of human sexuality through a biblical lens. It tackles difficult topics with grace, conviction, and hope—reminding us that if God calls us to sexual holiness, He also empowers us to pursue it. The book doesn't claim to be a counseling manual, yet it serves as a valuable tool for those walking alongside others in discipleship, marriage, or pastoral care. It helps put sexuality, desire, and identity back under God's authority—where they belong. For anyone longing to understand sexuality through the lens of Scripture, Pastor Jeff Schlenz speaks with truth, grace, and enduring relevance."

—Árpád Horváth Kávai, senior pastor at Calvary Chapel in Budapest (district 11), professor of pastoral psychology at Pentecostal Theological College in Budapest

"There has long been a need for a book on sexuality that combines the Bible's teaching with a shepherd's heart. Many books either diminish the Bible's plain teaching or convey an accusatory and judgmental tone. In *Authority over Attraction*, Pastor Jeff Schlenz avoids both of these errors. This book is firmly rooted in what the Bible says about sin and sex, yet Schlenz's tone is always pastoral. The discussion questions at the end of each chapter invite reflection, and the book itself draws its readers in. By the end, you will be thankful for the gift of the gospel—which not only saves but sanctifies us as well."

—Dr. Jesse Johnson, professor of theology at The Master's Seminary in Washington, DC

"From the perspective of a pastor and with the compassion of a shepherd, Jeff Schlenz delves into vital topics about God's design for our sexuality, offering insights that enlighten, challenge, and equip us in our spiritual growth."

—MARK RAMIREZ, senior pastor at
Calvary Chapel in Fredericksburg, VA

"*Authority over Attraction* is a much-needed book that I'm certain to use in ministry. This is a quick read on important issues that are grounded in Scripture. Pastor Jeff Schlenz, a longtime ministry partner, has done a great job of presenting biblical principles with care, firmness, and easy-to-follow logic. This is a book that everyone will benefit from—whether single or married, a parent or a grandparent—in seeking to understand what the Bible has to say about sexuality."

—TROY WARNER, senior pastor at
Calvary Chapel in Lynchburg, VA

Authority
over
Attraction

Authority
over
Attraction

*What Does God Say
About Sex and Sexuality?*

Jeff Schlenz

Authority over Attraction: What Does God Say About Sex and Sexuality?
Copyright © 2025 by Jeff Schlenz. All rights reserved.

Disclaimer: The views and opinions expressed in this book are those of the author and do not necessarily reflect the official policy or position of the United States Air Force, the Department of Defense, or the United States government.

Unless otherwise marked, Scripture is taken from the New King James Version®. Copyright © 1982 by Thomas Nelson. Used by permission. All rights reserved.

Scripture quotations marked (ESV) are from the ESV® Bible (the Holy Bible, English Standard Version®), © 2001 by Crossway, a publishing ministry of Good News Publishers. Used by permission. All rights reserved.

Thanks to:

GOOD ~~KARMA~~ Comma EDITING

for editing, interior layout, and cover design.
www.GoodCommaEditing.com

ISBN: 979-8-218-77405-9

Contents

Preface i

Introduction: Holy Sexuality 1

1. Sex Is a Gift, Not a God 13

2. Fully Known, Fully Loved: God's Good Design for Marital Intimacy 27

3. Passionate, Pleasant, and Pure 37

4. The Pitfall of Pornography 67

5. Against Nature: Submitting Sinful Desire to God's Authority 87

6. Escaping the Trap of Sexual Sin 111

7. The Source of Our Sexual Struggles 133

Appendix A: Common Questions and Answers 149

Appendix B: Recommended Resources 173

Preface

I did not want this to be my first book. Why? Because I don't want to be known as the guy who wrote a book on sex and sexuality. I want to be known as a guy who faithfully pastored a congregation and taught them God's Word. Unexpectedly, that's how I came to deal with this topic.

Early in my pastoral ministry, I was struck by the weight of being a pastor. This job is more than just preaching sermons about Jesus; it also involves helping people make big decisions as they apply Scripture to every area of their lives.

I still remember the first time a man came to me and asked if it was OK for him to get a vasectomy. I realized he was not just asking for another person's opinion; he was asking for his pastor's opinion . . . for God's opinion. For the rest of this man's life, whenever he would reflect on his decision, whether he did or did not get a vasectomy, part of the story he would tell himself and others would be, "Well, I talked with my pastor about it, and here's what he said."

The weight of that moment still sits with me today. It is why I originally wrote a booklet titled *Passionate,*

Pleasant, and Pure: A Biblical Look at Sex the Way God Intended. That booklet eventually became chapter 3 of this book.

In 2024, nearly fifteen years after I wrote the booklet, I was preaching through the book of Romans, which meant I had to address homosexuality. And I was addressing it at a time when transsexuality had become a prominent topic of discussion in our culture. In a single generation, sex and sexuality had shifted from the privacy of the bedroom to the top of our social media feeds, to public school curricula, and to displays in department stores.

My motivation with these sermons wasn't to seek conflict with the culture or have a sermon clip go viral; I simply aimed to move chapter by chapter, verse by verse, through whole books of the Bible, and that commitment had brought me into conflict with the culture. But to remain faithful to Scripture, I knew I had to address the issue of homosexuality directly.

As I prayed and thought about the best way to approach this topic, I determined that I would address all the ways we twist God's design for sex and sexuality to serve our own benefit and pleasure, regardless of the form that twisting takes. In other words, I would discuss other forms of sexual sin before addressing homosexuality so that we might all recognize how broken we are and not distract ourselves by pointing fingers at someone else's sin.

This choice meant I would also need to address the issue of pornography, which is a much more common trap for people today. Many Christians have had some experience with pornography in one form or another. This may simply mean that they heard about it and it aroused their curiosity but that in the end—by God's grace—they resisted that curiosity, avoided sin, and pressed further into Jesus.

For many others, though, it means their curiosity got the best of them. Whether they discovered it on their own or had someone else show it to them, they were pulled into sin. Some make a hasty retreat, having learned a lesson, and now praise God for keeping them from returning to it. But others fall in and cannot let go. They stay stuck, trapped, and unhappy in their sin. Of those trapped, some may hate it, but others have found a way to justify it to themselves, even though conviction still keeps them uncomfortable.

Then there are other individuals who are affected by a loved one's use of pornography. This is especially common in marital relationships, in which exposure to the fantasy world of pornography impacts a spouse's expectations and attraction to the person they pledged to remain faithful to for life.

As a pastor, I firmly believe that pornography poses one of the greatest threats to our spiritual health today. The question is, How do we respond to it?

I am (at the time of this book's publication) fifty years old. I attended church off and on for most of my life, though God really got ahold of me in 1997 when I was twenty-three years old, after I had my own experience with pornography as a young Marine living overseas.

In 2002, God called me into ministry. Maybe I missed something, and maybe I went to different churches, retreats, and conferences than you, but as my memory serves, pastors didn't talk about pornography from the pulpit back then. It may have come up at a men's retreat or in a private conversation, but pornography and sexual intimacy were not topics we expected to hear extensively addressed on Sunday morning.

But these topics need to be discussed, and we know this because Jesus and Paul spoke about them in the first century! The challenge is to take the right approach, remaining scripturally faithful without being lewd, provocative, or crude. This presented a significant pastoral challenge for me as I worked through Romans 1. Each Sunday, I wondered, *Is it OK for me to say this or that word from the pulpit? Are the senior saints and gospel grandparents going to be shocked and offended at what the pastor just said? Will parents be uncomfortable with me talking about this in front of their kids? Will I be comfortable talking about this in front of my own kids sitting in the sanctuary?* I usually felt a little awkward and nervous. It kept me in constant prayer, which is a good thing! But if God's Word clearly addresses a topic, and people are struggling with it, then we need to be able to shine the light of truth on it.

What you are about to read is an adaptation of those sermons preached at The City Gates Church during the fall of 2024 as I sought to be faithful to Scripture and avoid being unnecessarily explicit. The questions and answers in Appendix A are based on real questions I received from our congregation during and after the sermon series.

In other words, I didn't write this book to make a name for myself. I didn't write this book to confront cultural issues. I wrote this book to help people understand God's plan for their sex and sexuality, to help them see that His plan is best, and to encourage them to let go of anything that might be holding them back from that plan.

I hope this book is a blessing to you. I hope it stirs your affection for Christ. I hope it helps you confront any

Preface

sexual sin and temptation in your life and enables you to care for and minister to others in Jesus's name.

> No temptation has overtaken you except such as is common to man; but God is faithful, who will not allow you to be tempted beyond what you are able, but with the temptation will also make the way of escape, that you may be able to bear it.
>
> —1 Corinthians 10:13

Introduction: Holy Sexuality

In this book, we're going to take on subjects like pornography, adultery, homosexuality, and premarital sex. We're going to look at what God has to say about whom we sleep with and what we do in our bedrooms. It may be awkward and uncomfortable at times, but my goal is to point your heart toward Jesus, the source of satisfaction and joy. By embracing what the Bible teaches about sexuality, I pray you will grow closer to God, becoming more satisfied in who He is, what He is doing, and why He has made us. I hope that if God is calling you to give something up, you will do it by faith, believing that you will gain even more.

Perhaps a God-honoring sexuality was your goal at some point in the past, but you have fallen into temptation and sin along the way. Maybe you have become cynical and tired from trying and failing to live by God's holy standard. If that is your story, I pray that God will grant you the mustard-seed faith and desire to call out to Him, get back up, and try again, believing that He really can and will help you change.

I believe all of this is attainable, because it's all offered through Jesus. It's what we were meant to have. Paul writes in 1 Thessalonians 4:3, "For this is the will of God, your sanctification: that you should abstain from sexual immorality." If God wills us to walk in sexual holiness, He can surely empower us to do it.

Why I Wrote This Book

If God's will for our sexuality is so clear in Scripture, why write an entire book about it? I'll give you four reasons.

1. Sexuality is a big deal.

These days, subjects like sexual conduct and gender identity seem to be up for debate, even among Christians. Yet they're not things we can agree to disagree about in order to get along. Romans 1 clearly communicates that this is a first-tier issue: *sexual sin has eternal consequences*. That warning is repeated in passages like 1 Corinthians 6:9–10:

> Do you not know that the unrighteous will not inherit the kingdom of God? Do not be deceived. Neither fornicators, nor idolaters, nor adulterers, nor homosexuals, nor sodomites, nor thieves, nor covetous, nor drunkards, nor revilers, nor extortioners will inherit the kingdom of God.

Of the ten sins listed here, four of them have to do with sexuality. It's important to note that there's no bias or discrimination; Paul lumps together homosexuals and heterosexuals and says *they're both condemned*. Sex and sexuality are a really big deal, and eternity is at stake.

2. This is a discipleship issue.

These subjects are prominent in our culture, our families, and our churches. Sexual sin is not just something *they* deal with *out there*; it's something that happens in our own hearts, in our own homes, and in our own congregations. Sexual sin affects all kinds of people: men and women, young and old. Neither marriage nor advancing age exempts us; you don't "grow out of" the potential for temptation. So, we all need to know what God says about sexuality and how to respond to the ideas, images, and impulses that come into our minds.

And if this isn't you—if sexual desires and temptations have never been a challenge for you, or if this is a dragon you've already conquered—I hope this book will equip you to minister to others. In 2 Corinthians 1:3–4, Paul reminds us that we can take the comfort we receive from God and use it to comfort others in their distress. Imagine churches full of people who are competent to counsel in this issue, helping their kids, siblings, friends, and coworkers think clearly about these things *and overcome them* through the gift of the gospel. Whom does God want to reach through you? Whom can you help?

3. This is a relationship issue.

Obviously, your sexuality affects your relationship with God. It also affects your relationship with your spouse, if you have one. But have you ever thought about how the choices you make regarding your sexual behaviors may affect your relationship with your kids and even your grandkids?

The impact of sexual sin can be multigenerational, because your inability to control yourself sexually may impact whether you even have kids or whether your marriage stays intact. One day, your kids may have to try to explain to their kids why Grandma and Grandpa aren't together: "Well, they were married at one point when I was your age, but after putting up with his pornography use for three years, she finally kicked him out." If that day ever came, I don't think you would say that satisfying your sexual urges was worth it.

Beyond that, there may be more subtle effects of sexual sin, such as the way it shapes how you regard and respond to people of the opposite sex. The attitudes and behaviors we exhibit regarding gender and sexuality are learned by our children, who will then pass down many of those lessons to their children. The aftershocks of sexual sin can be felt for decades.

4. This is a gospel issue.

After listing ten sins in 1 Corinthians 6:9–10 that lead to divine condemnation, Paul says something crucial for our victory over sexual sin:

> And such were some of you. But you were washed, but you were sanctified, but you were justified in the name of the Lord Jesus and by the Spirit of our God. (1 Corinthians 6:11)

Here's the good news: Your past doesn't have to trap you or define you. Jesus can make *anyone* clean.

The Christian faith celebrates transformation. The gospel shows us that it's OK not to be OK—but it's not

Introduction: Holy Sexuality

OK to stay that way. Once we grasp the bad news that we have sinned against a holy God and deserve His righteous wrath, then we're ready for the truly good news that Jesus Christ died and rose again as a substitutionary sacrifice to remove our sin and clothe us in His own righteousness!

General Principles

I recognize addressing the issue of sexuality can be difficult. The truths in the following pages will be hard to read at times. They may cut close and feel personal. So I want to share some general principles up front to help you hear what I'm saying and understand where I'm going with this.

1. My goal is to draw you in, not push you out.

I can't sit here and tell you all your sexual impulses and experiences are acceptable and praiseworthy. I will not downplay your sin or its consequences. But I want to address these issues with both clarity and kindness, truth and grace, justice and mercy. Jesus said hard things, but sinners still came to hear Him because He loved them by telling them the truth.

2. I'm writing as a pastor.

I'm not a professor presenting a paper at a seminar. I'm not an expert in all the finer points of these issues. I'm also not a therapist addressing your specific circumstances. One of the greatest challenges of writing about this subject is trying to address a large audience of people with diverse circumstances. I might not address your specific situation very well. That's OK; the Word of God reveals what's true for everyone, regardless of their past or present. *Don't assume you're the exception to what is true for everyone else.*

I'm also not a politician seeking to address public policy; I know what the law of the land says about these issues. Instead, I'm here as an ambassador of the Kingdom of God to tell you what Scripture says, no matter where you land personally.

3. Distinctions matter.

If you're going to understand these issues well, you need to know there's a difference between temptation and sin. There is a line between impulse and behavior. You can be tempted without sinning. That's what happened to Jesus in the desert after His baptism.

Scripture says it like this:

> For we do not have a High Priest who cannot sympathize with our weaknesses, but was in all points tempted as we are, *yet without sin*. (Hebrews 4:15, emphasis mine)

When you have an intrusive thought or a sudden memory of past sin, you're being tempted, but you have not committed sin at this point. Sin requires intent and action. We absolutely must hold on to this distinction, because while God rightly judges our sin, He sympathizes with us in our weakness and temptation and, as we will see, helps us to resist.

For Christians, there is also an important distinction between *conviction* and *condemnation*. Both occur after

Introduction: Holy Sexuality

we've sinned, but they come from two different sources and lead in two different directions.

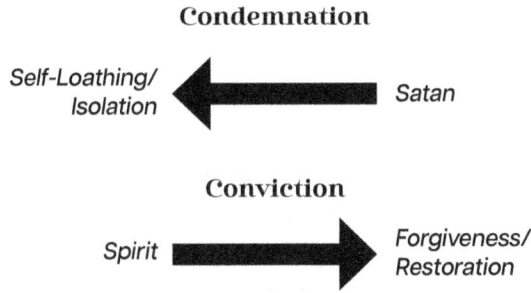

In the life of the believer, condemnation is soul-crushing, self-defeating negativity that comes from Satan, whom Scripture describes as our accuser. Condemnation drives us away from God to sulk in our shame and focus on our failure. But for all believers, condemnation is a lie. "There is therefore now no condemnation to those who are in Christ Jesus," as Paul says (Romans 8:1).

Conviction, on the other hand, comes from the Holy Spirit. The Spirit also says what we've done is wrong, but He turns our gaze away from ourselves and toward Jesus to find forgiveness and restoration.

When you read the Bible, you don't find Jesus crushing people caught in sexual sin. He's often hard on the self-righteous, but to people stuck in their sin—prostitutes, adulterers, the sexually immoral—He is gentle and merciful, offering forgiveness and a way out.

If you feel a sense of shame about your actions and choices, do not let it drive you away from God; instead, let it push you toward Him. Don't go around moping about your weakness. Don't believe the lie that you can never be forgiven. You were made for more than this, and you can overcome it.

4. You *can* change.

Maybe you have struggled with sexual temptation and failure for years, and you wonder deep down if God can actually change you. I'm here to tell you that He can and He will. God does not want to leave you as a slave to sin and sexual brokenness. The same gospel that saves your soul will set you free from this sin—maybe not freedom from the *temptation itself* (at least, in this life) but freedom from the slavish control of sin that causes you to act on that temptation. God doesn't want you half saved; He wants you to be set free and filled with faith, love, and truth. But here's the thing: That transformation might look like a miracle, or it might look like a mud run.

I ran my first mud run at Camp Pendleton in Southern California long before Spartan races were popularized. It was a ten-kilometer race, involving more than six miles of running over, under, and through all sorts of obstacles, including deep, sticky mud. We literally duct-taped our shoes to our feet so they didn't come off in the muck. By the end of the race, most runners were covered with dirt and mud from head to toe. Still, you couldn't wipe the smile off each finisher's face if you tried. It was a challenge, but that's why we felt so good after it was over: We did it!

When it comes to your fight with sexual temptations and sins, God might miraculously pick you up, clean you off, and set you down six miles later. More likely, though, He will lead you through six miles of sweat, struggle, and strain. You may stumble and fall. You may

Introduction: Holy Sexuality

backslide. You may need to repent of the same kinds of sin over and over again. All throughout, you may wish God would make it easy for you. That's not a bad wish. But for most people, it's going to be hard. That's OK. God is walking with you, and people are ready to help you. By God's grace and with His strength, *you can change.*

You're not so lost that He can't find you.

You're not so broken that He can't fix you.

You're not so dirty that He can't cleanse you.

Jesus specializes in rescue, renewal, and restoration—if you will surrender to Him. God has a better plan for your sexuality. Surrender it, as well as every other part of your life, to Him.

Reflection Questions – Introduction

1. Reflect on Romans 1:24–27. What are the ways in which you might be tempted to suppress God's truth in your own life? How can you seek to overcome these tendencies?

2. How do you personally understand the difference between temptation and sin, as outlined in the chapter? Share a specific example of a temptation you've faced and how you navigated it.

3. Sexual sin can have an impact on relationships and future generations. How might your current actions or attitudes toward sexuality affect your relationships with others, including your family?

4. How can your local church support individuals who are struggling with sexual temptation or sin while maintaining a balance of truth and grace? What practical steps can be taken to create a supportive environment?

5. How can a deeper theological understanding of God's design and purpose for sexuality enhance your faith and relationships?

6. Consider the four reasons given for addressing sexual issues: its significance and its discipleship, relational, and gospel implications. How do these reasons resonate with you, and which one do you find most compelling or challenging?

7. In this book, we will seek to see sexuality through the lens of God's authority and good design. How can you practically apply this understanding in

Introduction: Holy Sexuality

your everyday life, and what might it look like to offer your sexuality as a gift to God?

1

Sex Is a Gift, Not a God

We live in a confused culture that argues that sex is both everything and nothing.

Sex is everything. No one can suppress it, deny it, or tell you what you cannot do with it. Sex and sexuality must be liberated, set free from all boundaries. You are your sexuality, and your sexuality is you; your identity and self-understanding are fundamentally a product of your sexual expression. That concept touches everything from transgenderism to homosexuality to the need for "unrestricted access to contraception" and abortion (which are really two ways of saying the same thing).

In fact, the whole argument behind access to abortion is that if contraception didn't work or wasn't used before pregnancy, then terminating the life of an unborn child should be a suitable substitute for a condom or the pill. Why is abortion so important? Because if someone suppresses your sexuality or "punishes" you with a pregnancy that comes from having sex, that person "suppresses" you. That said, no one should dare suggest that you should limit your sexual expression to avoid that outcome. *Sex is everything—even if you have to kill for it.*

On the other hand, the message is also that *sex is nothing*. It doesn't really mean anything or do anything. It's no big deal. Therefore, there are no borders, no boundaries, and no restrictions. You don't need to be in a committed relationship or chained down in any way. You shouldn't expect the other person to be chained down to you, either. All that matters is consent, so if you're both in the mood, go for it. That's the enlightened and progressive approach to sex between consenting individuals.

The underlying contradiction is clear: *Sex cannot be everything and nothing at the same time.* Both ideas cannot be true. But this is the kind of convoluted situation we create when we suppress God's truth and ignore His boundaries. Instead of submitting our sexuality to Jesus, we make a god out of it. We submit to sex and let it run our life, and then we try to create a new moral law (like the ever-changing standards of "consent") to serve it.

When we do that, sex begins to undo us. It begins to reverse everything we were made for. Instead of bringing two parties together as one or creating new life, the infernal god of free sex keeps us from truly knowing our sexual partners and demands that we destroy any new life formed from the sexual act. After all, my sexuality says this is all about me, my desires, and my wants.

I suspect this is why sexual desolation is pictured in Romans 1 as emblematic of a person given over to their own desires. Allowing yourself to be driven by your impulses and urges ultimately drives you away from God and others.

One of the common arguments people make when they want to step outside of God's prescription for holy sexuality is that they cannot help whom they are attracted to or how strong that attraction is. It's as if attraction is a kind of unstoppable force like gravity, a law of the universe that cannot be denied or ignored. This deadly fiction has been woven into culture for generations, especially through media and the arts.

It should not be surprising that people feel driven by their attractions. In Romans 1:24, Paul writes that after mankind rejected the true God and began worshipping created things, they were given up to "uncleanness, in the lusts of their hearts, to dishonor their bodies among themselves." Later, Paul describes this as being given up to "vile passions" (Romans 1:26). In other words, when our worship became corrupted, our desires became warped. We began to want things that are destructive to us. This misshapen sexuality is characteristic of those who suppress God's truth and are given over to judgment. This is why sexuality should be understood primarily as an issue of *authority*, not *attraction*. Authority is the principle that determines the Christian view of sex and sexuality.

Authority Before Attraction

When people come to me facing sinful temptation, I am never interested in discussing who or what they are attracted to or how strong their desires are. I don't doubt any of those things; even pastors experience attractions and desires! The thing I want to know, more than anything else, is whose authority they are under. Sexuality is always an issue of authority before it becomes an issue of attraction. It's about what we believe, not what we feel.

When I feel an impulse, an urge, or a sense of excitement or arousal, who or what determines whether that's something I should follow? Is it "my body, my choice"? Or is it "You shall not commit adultery" (Exodus 20:14)? Do I determine my own truth and ethics, or does someone or something outside me tell me what I should pursue and what I should deny? You're going to go along with someone. The question is, Which voice is loudest in your mind?

- It might be your own voice. Once puberty hits, we all start to wake up sexually, and we have certain drives, impulses, and interests. What will you do with them? Do you follow whatever desire enters your head, or do you put boundaries around those desires?

- Do you allow your boyfriend or girlfriend or current hookup to determine what's OK? When they pressure you, invite you, or lure you to do things, do you go along or resist?

- Do you listen to the culture, allowing it to mold you and tell you what your sexual boundaries or expectations should be?

- Do you let your friends pressure you? Do they get to decide what you should be doing?

Someone will be the authority over your sexual life. Someone will set the standard and determine what is OK and what is not. Someone will make the rules. The Bible teaches that the one who determines the boundaries of your life is actually the God who created both you and sexual intimacy. Why not go by the manufacturer's instructions?

If sexual sin is called out in Romans 1 as the apex of suppressing truth and resisting God, our goal should be to repent (or turn around) and to bring sex and sexuality back under His authority. When we do that, we can accept and embrace what God reveals about sex, recognizing that He is the only authority over our sexual interests and activities. Our standard of truth is not our urges and impulses, not the pressures of our friends or a boyfriend or girlfriend, and not the pressures of our culture. God alone is our standard for truth.

Submitting to the lordship of Jesus Christ is the ultimate goal of life. We must bring every aspect of our lives under His authority—including our sexuality. By God's grace and with His strength, we must resist temptation on all fronts; this is a battle God wants to help us win. He doesn't just cheer for us; He instructs, equips, and strengthens us for the effort.

We need to bring all of our impulses, ideas, and feelings to God and say, "I will serve You, not these. I will serve You, not my anxiety. I will serve You, not my anger. I will serve You, not my pride. I will serve You, not my greed." This will happen when we submit to what God has revealed and refuse to suppress the truth.

Celebrating God's Good Gift of Sex

As we submit to God's authority over all aspects of life, we also need to understand that God is not only sovereign—He is also *good*. He sets boundaries, but He sets them in "pleasant places" (Psalm 16:6). There are reasons for the things He says yes to and the things He says no to.

Authority over Attraction

We often forget this clear and obvious fact: *God invented sex.* That seems so basic, but we need the reminder. We typically don't want to think theologically about sex. But the fact of the matter is that God designed the boy parts and the girl parts, and He made them to go together. God is the one who determined that sex was the way men and women were going to make babies, and He also determined that it would be enjoyable. God commanded Adam and Eve in Genesis 1:28 to "be fruitful and multiply," which essentially means, "Go, make *lots* of babies." As scandalous as it may sound at first, it's right and proper to give God the praise He deserves: He invented sex, and He made it fun. Glory to His name!

So, take a moment and think about sex theologically. (You probably think about it enough on your own; I'm just asking you to think about it in light of God's goodness!) Everything good that you enjoy about intimacy was made possible by God. He didn't have to give you those nerve endings in those places. He didn't have to design you to react the way you do and feel the things you do. In other words, it's not essential to existence or even to reproduction for you to *enjoy* being aroused. But you do enjoy it, *because God designed you that way*. He gave you that capacity as a gift. He wanted to bless you.

Many years ago, I had a slice of cheesecake from a place in New Jersey that was so good, it led me to fast from eating as an act of worship to God. Here's why: As I was eating that delicious, creamy slice of dessert with a thick graham cracker crust and caramel and apple woven into it, I realized that the only reason I could enjoy it is because God gave me taste buds. He didn't have to! God could have designed our digestive processes in a purely functional way, without regard to flavor or aroma. We just need calories and nutrients, and we can get them in many ways, like by chewing bamboo as a panda would. But God gave us the capacity to taste and to enjoy what we eat! He made a world full of flavor and spice and aroma that adds to our enjoyment of His creation and leads us to worship Him.

Friends, God gave us the capacity to enjoy His very good world, to experience delight and pleasure, including sensual pleasure. We might misuse the gift, but the gift itself, the original capacity, was put in place by the generous, joyous, and gracious God who loves us.

People talk about sex and sexuality all the time, and God is almost always left out of the conversation. Even among Christians, we don't often reflect on His role in our sexuality. If anything, we just reflect on His rules—and sometimes that's in order to avoid them or get around them. But if you're living under God's authority and following His commands, you should be able to praise Him for the pleasures you experience, even sexual pleasures. In fact, we might even go so far as to say that everything good that you enjoy about sexuality and arousal was designed by God, *and you may not be giving Him the glory for it that He truly deserves!*

Considering sex in the light of God's generous provision helps us understand that God really does have a good plan and purpose for us. Not only does He give us an appetite, but He also wants to guide us in how best to satisfy it. As we see more clearly how good God is, we may become more open to trusting Him and living within the boundaries He has established.

Know the Boundaries

The biblical boundaries of holy sexuality are simple to define: *celibacy outside of marriage and chastity within it.* That means your sexuality is to be shared only with one person: the person to whom you make a lifelong, covenantal commitment.

The best analogy I have ever heard for this is that of a fire in a fireplace. People are drawn to the warmth and comfort of a fire. It's so relaxing and soothing that many of us have gas fireplaces in our homes so that we can make it look and feel like we've got a fire going with just the flip of a switch. Even if you don't have a fireplace, you can go online and find videos with a continuous loop of logs burning, complete with the occasional crackle and snap.

Fire is also a useful tool. Several winters ago, we lost power in a large storm, but I was able to build a fire in the fireplace in our living room, rig a sling to hold a pot, and boil water. We made coffee and oatmeal and huddled near the hearth for warmth. That fire made our lives better when we needed it.

But what happens if you move that exact same fire two feet outside the fireplace and into the living room? Disaster. You still have flames. You still have heat. You still have crackling. But now it's coming from the couch, and that's not good.

In this analogy, we see two very different ways to experience the same gift. Fire can be good, enjoyable, and helpful when it is kept in its rightful place, but it can be devastating, destructive, and all-consuming when it is not. Sex inside the covenant of marriage is beautiful, but sex outside of marriage is detrimental.

Now consider this: The destructive fire of taking sex outside of God's boundaries can take various forms. It can start "inside the house" if you look at sexually explicit images alone in your room. It can come from "outside the house" with a spark of a flirtation with someone who is not your spouse. Either way, when we play with fire that is not contained by the fireplace, it will lead to destruction. That's why King Solomon uses similar imagery to warn his son (and us) against the dangers of sexual sin:

> Can a man take fire to his bosom, and his clothes not be burned? Can one walk on hot coals, and his feet not be seared? So is he who goes in to his neighbor's wife; whoever touches her shall not be innocent. (Proverbs 6:27–29)

Playing with Matches

Unmarried readers may see the reference to adultery in this Proverbs passage and assume it does not apply to them. Do not be deceived; any sexual activity before or outside of marriage is just as dangerous as adultery during marriage. We will talk about pornography in chapter 4, but let me take a moment to talk about hookup culture: the attempt to normalize sex without commitment. We already know that Scripture says we should practice celibacy outside of marriage and maintain chastity within marriage. Now, science is saying the same thing: Recent studies in neuroscience align with the truth of God's Word.

Dr. Joe Malone holds a PhD in health and human performance with a minor in neuropsychology and a specialization in women's health and sexual wellness.

He has been a professor and guest lecturer at several schools, including Vanderbilt and Princeton.

Dr. Malone's research has produced interesting findings on the damaging aspects of a casual attitude toward sex. He has found that the faster sexual intimacy enters a relationship, the less likely the relationship is to last. He explains this phenomenon in neurological terms that I'm not smart enough to summarize, but basically it takes at least four months of an exclusive relationship between a man and a woman before sufficient attachment has been formed in the man's brain that leads him to want to remain in the relationship. If a couple rushes to sexual intimacy before at least those four months of nonsexual emotional bonding, their connection will not properly establish in the man's brain, and neither will his sense of commitment. The research shows that the relationships in which sexual intimacy is achieved most quickly also end the fastest.[1]

The rush toward sexual intimacy damages future relationships too. According to Malone's research and other studies from the National Institutes of Health, one of the top indicators of adultery and divorce in later relationships is the number of premarital partners a person has had. As that number goes up, the likelihood of a permanent, pure, lifelong marriage goes down.[2]

---

1. For an article by Dr. Malone with footnotes to relevant sources, see Joe Malone, "College Hookup Culture Pulls Women Out of the Driver's Seat When It Comes to Introducing Sex in Relationships," Natural Womanhood, February 24, 2023, https://naturalwomanhood.org/hookup-culture-in-college-hurts-young-women-the-most/.

2. Jesse Smith and Nicholas Wolfinger, "Re-Examining the Link Between Premarital Sex and Divorce," *Journal of Family Issues* 45, no. 3 (2023): 674–696, https://doi.org/10.1177/0192513x231155673.

It turns out that there really are consequences for those who misuse what God has created and who suppress the truth of His good design. You can kick and push against it all you want. You can deny and ignore it. You can make excuses for why you should be able to do it your way, but you can't completely disarm the consequences. When you go against the grain of the universe, you get splinters.

Remember, God never said we should not enjoy the fire. He just told us to keep it in the fireplace so we don't burn ourselves. Boundaries are good things.

Rather than chase the sexual high of serial hookups, God's best plan is for most men and women to get married and for sexual intimacy to be a part of that exclusive, lifelong commitment. God's best plan is for both the man and the woman to be surrendered to each other, to enjoy and delight in each other, and to trust the loyalty of each other fully and completely. In God's best plan, the man and woman can be naked and unashamed (Genesis 2:25) so that the marriage bed is undefiled (Hebrews 13:4). When we follow God's blueprint, there are no regrets, and there is no baggage.

At this point, some of you may be feeling that sense of condemnation welling up within you—especially if you have a history of "playing with matches." Let me remind you again that Jesus Christ died for sinners like you and me, not just to pay the penalty for our sins but also to cleanse us from all unrighteousness. All your regrets and baggage can be forgiven and redeemed in Christ. No matter your sexual background or the mistakes you have made, if you are ready to repent of your sexual sin, Jesus stands ready to make you clean. You can put the matches down and walk in the light again. And if you have already repented of this sin from your past and know Christ as your Savior, know that you are not condemned. You are not a slave to this sin anymore, and it does not define you. You have been washed, sanctified, and justified in the name of Jesus (1 Corinthians 6:11).

Reflection Questions – Chapter 1

1. What are some common challenges or pressures that make it difficult for you to submit your sexuality to Jesus? How can you overcome these challenges with God's help?

2. How do you personally respond to the idea that sexuality is a reflection of your rebellion against, or alignment with, God?

3. In what ways does our culture influence our understanding and practice of sexuality? How can we discern and resist cultural pressures that conflict with God's design?

4. What are some specific ways that your friends, the media, or societal expectations have influenced your views and behaviors regarding sexuality? How can you evaluate and adjust these influences to better align with God's truth?

5. How can studying Scripture and seeking God's wisdom help you better understand and appreciate His design for sexuality? What specific passages or teachings have been particularly impactful in shaping your view?

6. When faced with sexual temptation, how can you remind yourself that God's authority should guide your actions? What practical strategies can help you stay aligned with His guidance?

2

Fully Known, Fully Loved: God's Good Design for Marital Intimacy

When a man and woman who are committed to walking in holy sexuality decide to covenant together in marriage, they experience a sexual relationship in which they can be fully known and fully loved. Ironically, Christians typically use that kind of language in light of the gospel, to convey the idea that God knows everything about you and loves you anyway. In Christ, you are fully known and fully loved. But Scripture uses similar language when it makes the first reference to sexual intercourse; it's described as a man *knowing* his wife. One benefit of knowing and living within God's boundaries for sexuality is that you get the joy and privilege of knowing your spouse fully and freely.

Knowing Your Spouse

The Bible uses this language of *knowing* several times when referencing sexual intimacy:

> Now Adam *knew* Eve his wife, and she conceived and bore Cain, and said, "I have acquired a man from the LORD." (Genesis 4:1, emphasis mine)

And Cain *knew* his wife, and she conceived and bore Enoch. (Genesis 4:17, emphasis mine)

And Elkanah *knew* Hannah his wife, and the LORD remembered her. (1 Samuel 1:19, emphasis mine)

In Judges 11:39, a virgin is described as someone who "*knew* no man" (emphasis mine). Mary, the mother of Jesus, responded to the angelic announcement in this way: "How can this be, since I do not *know* a man?" (Luke 1:34, emphasis mine).

In some of these contexts, different translations of the Bible tend to flatten the meaning of the Hebrew word that the New King James Version renders as "know":

- New International Version: "made love"

- New American Standard Bible: "had relations"

- New Living Translation: "had sexual relations," "slept with"

But the Hebrew word used in these contexts, *yadah*, actually means "to know, to perceive, to discriminate or distinguish, or to know by experience." Sexual intercourse is an expression of intimacy, but something more than physical is happening. The Bible says two are becoming one (Genesis 2:24), and something powerful is being learned. There is a knowledge and experience of each other that no one else is ever meant to discover or share.

Here's what that means for our discussion of holy sexuality: You are made to be fully known and fully loved, first by the God who made you and knows your every thought and also by the spouse to whom you have promised your lifelong faithfulness. Sexual intimacy, within the bounds of marriage, is one way you know and are known by that man or woman. My friends, this is God's good, good plan!

The problem is, instead of accepting God's good plan for sex, people suppress the truth by rejecting their primary relationship with the God who knows them best and by filling His place in their lives with sex itself. Sex is an incredible gift—but it makes a terrible god.

Marital Intimacy Is a Ministry, Not a Buffet

Let me add a word of warning here for those of us who think we stand firm on this issue, lest we fall. It is tempting to look out at the world and be glad we are not like *those people* making sex their god—people who worship their sexuality and who are driven and defined by it. But Paul warns his religiously minded readers in Romans 2 not to be quick to condemn those who sin in such ways without also examining themselves.

You see, sexual sin is a tricky, devious, conceited little demon. It can put on a religious mask and use pious language, while secretly you worship it in your heart. This happens when, instead of worshipping God by submitting your sexuality to Him, you defer that worship to your sexual satisfaction with your spouse. Think of the unmarried Christian saying, "I can't wait to get married so I can finally have all the sex I want and won't have to struggle with lust." Here's the problem with this way of thinking: It's still all about them and their urges and desires. This person's experience, at the level of desire and motive, is no different than the most sex-saturated unbeliever. Sex is still in control; they're just trying to worship it in a "better" place. They imagine their future spouse as the buffet upon which they can satisfy their ravenous appetite. They look forward to the day when they can use their spouse for their selfish desires, with the sanction of a marriage certificate.

But the reality is, your spouse might not always be eagerly available to satisfy your sexual needs. Even if your spouse deeply cares for you, there will be times when they cannot be available sexually due to travel, illness, injury, and so on. That is why we are to strengthen our sexual self-control before marriage; we will need to exercise those muscles at various times and seasons during marriage. Paul writes this to the Thessalonians:

> For this is the will of God, your sanctification: that you should abstain from sexual immorality; that each of you should know *how to possess his own vessel in sanctification and honor, not in passion of lust*, like the Gentiles who do not know God; that no one should take advantage of and defraud his brother in this matter, because the Lord is the avenger of all such, as we also forewarned you and testified. For God did not call us to uncleanness, but in holiness. (1 Thessalonians 4:3–7, emphasis mine)

Even within the bounds of marriage, our sexual desires should be submitted to the will of Christ and dedicated to serving our spouse and not just ourselves. If you rely on your spouse's sexual availability as the only means to keep yourself in check, what do you do when your spouse is unable to support you? Do you make them feel guilty or pressured into what should be the defining act of intimacy in your marriage, just because you can't control yourself? What kind of burden are you putting on them? Is your husband or wife supposed to put your sinful flesh to death for you, or is that your job? It may be that some of us need to repent to God and to our spouse for putting the burden of our sanctification (and the blame for our lack of it) on them, rather than seeking to control our own bodies better. When we let sex, even marital sex, become our idol, we sacrifice true intimacy with our spouse in the process.

Healthy sexuality in Christian marriage is found in the tension between two truths: Spouses should be available to each other, and they should honor each other. Consider the words of Paul in 1 Corinthians 7 regarding being available to each other:

> Let the husband render to his wife the affection due her, and likewise also the wife to her husband. The wife does not have authority over her own body, but the husband does. And likewise the husband does not have authority over his own body, but the wife does. Do not deprive one another except with consent for a time, that you may give yourselves to fasting and prayer; and come together again so that Satan does not tempt you because of your lack of self-control. (1 Corinthians 7:3–6)

Christian husbands and wives should be willingly and happily available to their spouses for marital intimacy because their body belongs to their spouse. Abstaining from intimacy should be by mutual consent and for the sake of additional fasting and prayer. Intimacy should never be withheld as a punishment or offered as a tool of manipulation.

Also, Christian spouses should honor each other.

> Wives, submit to your own husbands, as to the Lord. For the husband is head of the wife, as also Christ is head of the church; and He is the Savior of the body. Therefore, just as the church is subject to Christ, so let the wives be to their own husbands in everything. Husbands, love your wives, just as Christ also loved the church and gave Himself for her, that He might sanctify and cleanse her with the washing of water by the word, that He might present her to Himself a glorious church, not having spot or wrinkle or any such thing, but that she should be holy and without blemish. (Ephesians 5:22–27)

Wives, what is your driving impulse as you view your husband? Are you submitting to him as the church submits to Christ? Husbands, what is your driving impulse as you view your wife? Are you hoping to sanctify her, cleanse her, and sacrifice yourself for her? Or are you asking her merely to be an outlet for your urges and desires? Are you truly loving her when you say you're "making love" to her? Are you honoring each other with your intimacy?

I want to say again that our sexual desires can be good *if* they are properly shaped and formed. They are a powerful impulse and urge to point us toward our spouse and the relationships we are meant to have with God and with each other. Desire can be a blinking light on the dashboard of our lives that tells us to go spend time with our spouse and be fully known and fully loved.

And if you're single, that drive is telling you to go find a spouse. Do not try to find a "soulmate" in the romantic movie sense, which is based on attraction and emotion instead of reality. Seek someone who loves Jesus like you do and who can do life with you. Look for a relationship in which you can help each other on the path to holiness, not just by satisfying sexual desire but by being fully known and fully loved.

Don't make a sad, shameful little god out of sex. Don't take it upon yourself to satisfy all your desires and don't shackle anyone else with those burdens either. If you make a god out of sex, it will never satisfy you. Only God is able to provide ultimate, enduring satisfaction—way down deep at the level of our soul. And only He is worthy of our submission and worship.

Our True Source of Satisfaction

Consider the testimony of Scripture and listen to those who have found true, durable, lasting satisfaction in God:

> O God, You are my God; early will I seek You; my soul thirsts for You; my flesh longs for You in a dry and thirsty land where there is no water. So I have looked for You in the sanctuary, to see Your power and Your glory. (Psalm 63:1–2)

> Whom have I in heaven but You? And there is none upon earth that I desire besides You. My flesh and my heart fail; but God is the strength

of my heart and my portion forever. (Psalm 73: 25–26)

The L ORD will guide you continually, and satisfy your soul in drought, and strengthen your bones; You shall be like a watered garden, and like a spring of water, whose waters do not fail. (Isaiah 58:11)

On the last day, that great day of the feast, Jesus stood and cried out, saying, "If anyone thirsts, let him come to Me and drink. He who believes in Me, as the Scripture has said, out of his heart will flow rivers of living water." (John 7:37–38)

Imagine that: You are thirsty, driven by desire, so you come to Jesus, who doesn't just fill you but fills you until you overflow. You are wholly and completely satisfied in the God who made you.

This is the life you were made for. This is what your life can be. You don't have to be driven by your sexuality or by the sexual desires of someone else. God gave you gender and sexuality, and they are good gifts to be used within proper boundaries. Sexual intimacy enables you to know and to be known in an exclusive, permanent covenant by someone who loves God and loves you. This is the great joy of submitting your sexuality to God rather than turning it into your god.

Maybe you've made a mess of things by trying to look out for yourself, scheming and conniving to get what you want. There is nothing you have done and nothing that has been done to you that God doesn't know about. You have no thoughts or desires that He doesn't know already. And yet, you're never too dirty for Jesus.

If you have turned sexual satisfaction into an idol, you can be forgiven and cleansed. If you are still struggling to walk in holiness and submit to authority rather than attraction, you can repent. You can receive what God reveals instead of suppressing the truth. You can walk in the Spirit instead of the flesh. You can move toward God's blessings instead of His wrath. You can confess, repent of your sin, submit your sexuality to Jesus, and let God give you what you need.

So talk to Him. Ask for forgiveness and strength. Ask for healing from the wounds of others. Ask to be made new, to be made holy. Whatever you need, ask God for it. He is ready to restore what is broken.

Reflection Questions – Chapter 2

1. According to this chapter, how should sexual intimacy be viewed within marriage? What are some ways couples can cultivate a healthy, God-centered approach to their sexual relationship? What are practical steps to practice celibacy and manage sexual desires before marriage?

2. How does the concept of "knowing" your spouse extend beyond physical intimacy to emotional and spiritual dimensions? How can couples work toward a deeper understanding and connection with each other?

3. How does being fully known and fully loved by God (Psalm 139:1–4; Romans 5:8) free us to love our spouses and others well despite their imperfections?

4. What practical steps can you take to foster deeper emotional and spiritual intimacy in your marriage or close relationships?

5. How can couples ensure that their sexual relationship enhances their marriage rather than becoming a source of conflict or unrealistic expectations? What are some healthy practices for fostering intimacy and mutual respect?

6. How does knowing that Christ alone fully satisfies (John 4:13–14) free us from unhealthy pursuits?

7. What are some practical ways to minister to your spouse emotionally, physically, and spiritually? How can prayer strengthen intimacy in marriage?

3

Passionate, Pleasant, and Pure

Not long ago, a man walked into my office and asked a courageous, honest question. He shared how his views on sex and sexuality had been broken for almost twenty years, but he said that it "worked" because it gave him what he wanted. Now, as he teetered on the edge of choosing to let go of what "worked" for him and embrace God's way, he wanted to know if he would still enjoy his sexuality.

I told him two things: that he needed to reassess and then retrain his appetite. For example, there is no doubt that we can physically crave foods that are terrible for us nutritionally. As a result, we might fill ourselves with "junk food" and lose our appetite for a good, grass-fed steak served alongside fresh greens and delicious, fresh fruit for dessert. The same applies to sexual appetite: One can indulge in unhealthy pursuits and lose interest in what is truly good and beautiful.

I said, "You need to reassess your appetite and ask yourself, 'While the things I consume may be "satisfying," are they healthy?' The answer is no. They're endangering you spiritually and threatening the future of your marriage, and they could one day destroy your career if you're discovered.

"But if you retrain your appetite, by God's grace and with His help, then yes, I assure you, God's ways are best. Remember, He has designed everything related to sexuality. It is a good, wholesome, and holy gift, and when we accept His terms, we will flourish."

So what does flourishing look like? What does healthy, holy sexuality look like—sexuality that is driven by our submission to God rather than our own attractions? What should we pursue? That's the focus of this chapter. There's a lot to discuss here, but my hope is that, regardless of who you are or what you're struggling with, you'll find something helpful in these pages.

The Blessing of Boundaries: Establishing Boundaries in Dating and Marriage

The boundaries for sexual interest and activities that we are about to discuss apply to both married and single people. Our actions, looks, and thoughts toward members of the opposite sex should be governed by holiness and purity, whether we are married or single. Paul gave Timothy specific instructions to treat "older women as mothers, younger women as sisters, with all purity" (1 Timothy 5:2).

In light of Paul's instructions, in every relationship we have, we are to love the other person innocently and with purity. There is no category for treating another image-bearer of God as "the tool that satisfies my sexual appetite."

Only Within the Walls of Marriage

The first step toward building a God-honoring view of sex is to understand where it belongs—which is within the walls of marriage.

> Therefore be imitators of God as dear children. And walk in love, as Christ also has loved us and given Himself for us, an offering and a sacrifice to God for a sweet-smelling aroma. But fornication and all uncleanness or covetousness, *let it not even be named among you*, as is fitting for saints; neither filthiness, nor foolish talking, nor coarse jesting, which are not fitting, but rather giving of thanks. For this you know, that no fornicator, unclean person, nor covetous man, who is an idolater, has any inheritance in the kingdom of Christ and God. Let no one deceive you with empty words, for because of these things the wrath of God comes upon the sons of disobedience. Therefore do not be partakers with them. (Ephesians 5:1–7, emphasis mine)

The word *fornication* in this passage is also translated as "sexual immorality" in some Bible versions. The word *porneia* is used for *fornication* in the Greek and refers to a variety of sexual activities outside the ethical boundaries of a marriage between one man and one woman.[1] That

---

1. Kenneth S. Wuest, *Wuest's Word Studies: Ephesians and Colossians in the Greek New Testament for the English Reader* (William B. Eerdmans Publishing, 1953), 120. Wuest says that "The word porneia was used of illicit sexual intercourse in general." Also see "porneia" in Wesley J. Perschbacher, *The New Analytical Greek Lexicon* (Hendrickson Publishers, 1990).

means the two criteria for appropriate sexual intimacy are that it takes place 1) within the bounds of marriage and 2) with one's spouse. Sex within the bounds of marriage, between one man and one woman, has always been God's plan; it is His wedding gift to every couple, meant to be enjoyed only after they exchange vows. It is not to be shared with anyone else before or during marriage.

Paul states that fornication, or any kind of sexual relationship outside of marriage, should "not even be named among you." It is entirely off-limits. In fact, he goes so far as to say that if your life is characterized by this sin, if you could rightly be called a "fornicator," you are under the wrath of God and have no inheritance in the Kingdom. There is forgiveness in Christ for those who repent of sexual sin, but the fornicator is someone who dwells in sin, feels comfortable there, and has no desire to change.

Only with Your Spouse

If God intends for sex to take place only within the bounds of marriage, that means it should be shared only with your spouse. This is the next step for building a God-honoring view of sex.

Not only has God forbidden premarital sex, but He has also prohibited sexual activity (whether actual or imagined) with anyone other than your spouse. Because sex outside of marriage is wrong, and because you should be married only to one person, this seems a bit obvious, but I've stated it nonetheless.

Lust is sinful coveting for another person, whether before or after marriage. It's even forbidden through one of the Ten Commandments:

> You shall not covet your neighbor's house; you shall not covet your neighbor's wife, nor his male servant, nor his female servant, nor his ox, nor his donkey, nor anything that is your neighbor's. (Exodus 20:17)

In His famous Sermon on the Mount, Jesus addressed this issue and went straight to the motive of the heart, as He often did:

> You have heard that it was said to those of old, "You shall not commit adultery." But I say to you that whoever looks at a woman to lust for her has already committed adultery with her in his heart. (Matthew 5:27–28)

Lusting after another person is mental robbery. You are seeking to pleasure yourself by having sexual thoughts about someone who already belongs, or will belong, with someone else. Further, you are neglecting your own current or future spouse by not receiving all of your delight from them. Wandering eyes and thoughts keep you from enjoying the spouse God has given to you.

How much better to say with Job, "I have made a covenant with my eyes; why then should I look upon a young woman?" (Job 31:1). The root of the Hebrew word used here for "look" is *bîn*. It is most often translated as "understand" or "consider." This is more than just noticing that someone is attractive; it's lingering, exploring, and interrogating them visually for one's own enjoyment.

The Bible actually has a lot to say on this subject. Read the words of Solomon in Proverbs 5:

Drink water from your own cistern, flowing water from your own well. Should your springs be scattered abroad, streams of water in the streets? Let them be for yourself alone, and not for strangers with you. Let your fountain be blessed, and rejoice in the wife of your youth, a lovely deer, a graceful doe. Let her breasts fill you at all times with delight; be intoxicated always in her love. Why should you be intoxicated, my son, with a forbidden woman and embrace the bosom of an adulteress? (Proverbs 5:15–20 ESV)

There should be only one outlet for all your sexual interest and energy throughout your life: your spouse. "Drink from your own cistern." Remember that God has established two main criteria for sexual intimacy: It is to occur only within the bounds of marriage and only with your spouse. Anything outside of these boundaries is a misuse of His gift.

Strengthening the Boundaries

The boundaries God has given us for enjoying sex are simple and for our protection, yet many believe the lie that they are unnecessarily restraining. These boundaries are under constant attack from the evil one: He tempts us from within to push against them while leading the world to do the same thing around us. They must be strengthened and defended constantly, or chips, cracks, and outright breaches will occur.

Much of what we typically see and much of what the Bible warns against relates to men lusting after women. However, women also need to be cautioned:

Do not seek love in the wrong places. We all know men typically struggle with physical desire, but women can experience the same impulse. Women must guard their hearts against longing for the men portrayed in movies and romance novels who appear more handsome, adventurous, courageous, mysterious, or sensitive than those in their own lives. Ultimately, temptation will take different forms for different people; the flesh and the Enemy of our souls are always searching for something to use to draw us outside of God's boundaries and away from finding complete and total satisfaction in His design for us.

Why is this such a big deal? It's because the marriage relationship illustrates Christ's relationship with the church. He has no other bride, and we should have no other husband. Because this is true spiritually, it must also be true in marriage.

Fortunately, God knows we live in a world that attacks us with temptation from every angle, and He is always there to help us live up to His standard. Consider His promise to us:

> No temptation has overtaken you except such as is common to man; but God is faithful, who will not allow you to be tempted beyond what you are able, but with the temptation will also make the way of escape, that you may be able to bear it. (1 Corinthians 10:13)

Know When to Start the Fire: A Word to Dating and Engaged Couples

Marriage is honorable among all, and the bed undefiled; but fornicators and adulterers God will judge.

—Hebrews 13:4

Unmarried couples often struggle with setting boundaries for their physical relationship, wondering, "How far can we go?" Before answering this question, let's consider the motive behind it. Is your desire to honor God with all your heart, soul, mind, and strength? And if so, are you asking how you can do that as you touch one another? Or are you asking, "How much of this can we enjoy before we say, 'I do'?"

The question should not be "How far can we go?" Instead, the question should be "When can we start?" The answer to both questions is this: "After you are married, you two can go as far as you want as often as you like!"

A fire can be a very useful and enjoyable thing when enjoyed within the boundaries of a fireplace, but if you simply move that fire two feet into the living room, you will cause a disaster. There is a proper time and place for the physical expressions of romantic love, but outside their boundaries, they become dangerous as well. Purity demands that the fire of a sexual relationship be kept within the fireplace of marriage.

In Song of Solomon, young ladies especially are encouraged to wait for love and romance until the proper time: "I charge you, O daughters of Jerusalem, do not stir up nor awaken love until it pleases" (Song of Solomon 8:4).

The problem is, we're like kids at Christmas who know there is this big present from God sitting under the tree, and we want to keep peeling back the corners of the wrapping paper to peek at what's inside instead of just waiting for December 25 to arrive.

You need to understand that it isn't "love" if someone asks or tempts you to do something that goes against God's will. If a guy or girl is tempting you to sin while dating—a time in which both people usually try to be on their best behavior—you should question if that person really respects you and cares about what's best for you. That could be a red flag for what your relationship will be like when the guardrails come down, whether it's before or after marriage. If that person doesn't respect you now, they won't respect you once you've given yourself to them physically. Instead, a godly couple should explore the possibility of a future in which both people truly love and want God's best for each other; neither should lead the other into sin. Do the raw ingredients of your relationship support this kind of future?

Purity will only become harder to maintain as you progress in your relationship. Your goal should be to "finish well." Like a marathon runner, you don't want to stumble in the last mile. Dive into Scripture, support and encourage each other, pray for each other, and ask God for the strength you need to finish the dating race well.

That said, if you are looking for a guide in establishing the boundaries of your physical relationship while dating, let me suggest that you never do anything in private that you wouldn't do in public. Nothing should be happening on the couch that you wouldn't want to be filmed and posted on your social media feed.

One of the best ways to protect your purity as a couple is to pray about it together. Ask God to watch over you in this regard. Agree together that this is something important that you want to protect. Establish the boundary line early in your relationship, discuss it, agree to it, and stick to it. I also recommend you write a contract explicitly stating where the boundary is and then sign it together. "Normal" relationships in our day and age race toward sexual intimacy; if you desire to honor both God and each other in your relationship, you will need to fight to be *abnormal*. What will you do? What steps will you take to protect yourselves against sliding into sexual sin? Make a plan together; then stick to it.

Dealing with the Past

Unfortunately, not everyone will enter marriage with the sexual purity God intended for them. Some fall intentionally; others are taken advantage of. The good news is that there is nothing that has been done by you or to you that Jesus cannot heal or restore. God's promise to the Israelites to "restore . . . the years that the swarming locust has eaten" (Joel 2:25) also applies to you. The Israelites experienced the consequences of wandering from God, but He was willing and able to restore what they lost if they returned to Him. My old pastor used to say, "God can restore your ability to blush." Whether you've intentionally wandered or have been taken advantage of, God can restore your innocence. There is nothing, absolutely nothing, that God cannot renew.

On another note, how much of your past sexual sin should you discuss with your spouse or fiancé? It is good to confess the fact that you have sinned sexually in the past, but should you share how many times you sinned this way and the details of those experiences? I don't think so.

There is little or nothing to be gained by such confessions, especially if Jesus has already forgiven those sins. My general rule is this: Discuss anything that is *still with you*. If there has been a history of abuse that could affect your ability to be intimate together, if you have children from a previous relationship, or if you have any form of STD, discuss it with your partner.[2]

Theology over Biology

Theology can always trump biology. No matter how strong the desire or temptation, God is always willing and able to help us defeat or escape it.

There are also practical steps you can take to help one another. Here are a few:

1. **Pray.** Pray for your spouse, that they would be protected from temptation, and that, when it comes, they would be strong enough in the Lord to resist it. Zealously protect your marriage and defend your spouse through prayer.

---

2. Depending on your background and experiences, as your relationship matures and becomes more serious, you may also want to share any situations or patterns that have been problematic for you. For example, you can share how, in certain situations, you have struggled with and/or given in to specific kinds of sexual temptation, such as pornography, hookups, and so on. Sharing these patterns can invite the other person into your pursuit of personal growth. They can pray for you and with you, help you avoid such temptations, and encourage you in your weaknesses.

2. **Reflect.** Identify your triggers. What is happening before you're tempted? What can you do to avoid those circumstances? Are you using sexuality to combat feelings of insecurity, boredom, or loneliness? Consider what may be the root of your sexual sin and how addressing it might correct some of your current behaviors. Seek help from the Lord and wise counsel for overcoming these issues before you fall into temptation.

3. **Engage.** Paul prescribes intimacy as a way to deflect the power of temptation:

> The husband should give to his wife her conjugal rights, and likewise the wife to her husband. The wife does not have authority over her own body, but the husband does. Likewise the husband does not have authority over his own body, but the wife does. Do not deprive one another, except perhaps by agreement for a limited time, that you may devote yourselves to prayer; but then come together again, *so that Satan may not tempt you because of your lack of self-control.* (1 Corinthians 7:3–5 ESV, emphasis mine)

A word of caution and clarification is necessary here. Self-control is also a fruit of the Spirit (Galatians 5:22–23). In other words, God is leading all Christians to grow in sexual self-control, with or without sexual release. There will be times when sexual intimacy is not available to spouses due to physical separation (e.g., business travel or military deployments) or medical concerns or illness. While the goal for intimacy is that it should be a regular and mutually enjoyed experience, both parties should be able to go through periods of Holy Spirit-enabled abstinence whenever necessary.

4. **Defend.** Watch what you let into your house and into your heart. Today, temptation can come through countless media—through our phones, our music, the books we read, or even the catalogs that come to us in the mail. As a couple, you will need to decide what you will allow into your home. Put the fences up wherever you need them, but do it together in agreement as a way to strengthen your marriage and please God.

The Purpose of Sex

What is the purpose of sex? If we can answer this question, many other questions will be answered as well. The act of making love can produce two possible positive results: an enjoyable, intimate experience of pleasure and the creation of children.

The question is, Should we pursue one end result more than the other? Is one more valid than the other? Is sex more for procreation or recreation? Is it primarily for having children, with enjoyment being an incentive to engage in it frequently enough to ensure reproduction actually takes place? Or should seeking enjoyment and intimacy be the primary pursuit in the bedroom?

Clearly, it is permissible to seek children through the act of intercourse; that's the only natural way they arrive biologically. But is it permissible to engage in intercourse without the primary intent being to have children? Yes, and for two reasons: First, look again at Paul's instruction to husbands and wives in 1 Corinthians 7:5. He tells them not to "deprive one another" and to "come together" to avoid being tempted because of their lack of self-control. This indicates that intercourse for the purpose of sexual fulfillment and intimacy within a marriage is both natural and acceptable. Second, biologically, God did not design women to be able to conceive every day. Therefore, it is possible (and even probable) that, most of the time, unprotected intercourse will *not* result in offspring.

Let us not forget who designed our bodies. It was God who placed all those nerve endings where He did, and it was God who designed arousal the way He did. He also created the menstrual cycle. God could have guaranteed that our reproductive systems would produce offspring each time, with pleasure and intimacy occurring only occasionally, but He didn't. Imagine that!

It seems clear, then, that He desired sexual intimacy to be an enjoyable experience for the couple, even when children are not conceived. Here we understand why the only appropriate context for sexual interaction is within the bounds of marriage: The depth of commitment in marriage is unmatched by any other human relationship we have.

Within the comforting and reassuring walls of this covenant, which we have made to each other in the sight of God, we are able to be completely exposed and to surrender ourselves entirely to each other. We engage in an experience that is so intimate that it is not shared with *anyone* except our spouse. In the marriage bed, we can give ourselves freely to someone who has promised they will never abandon us and will always stand by us. We bring pleasure to them and receive pleasure from them with trust, knowing we are not being used. Authentic sexual intimacy is a result of the trust established at the altar and found nowhere else.

So then, what is the purpose of sex? I propose this answer: Its purpose is to create an intimate experience of pleasure between a married man and woman, which they alone share and which may or may not produce offspring. Children are a possible, though not guaranteed, outcome of intercourse.

God-Glorifying Sex: Frequency and Form

One of the big questions men and women struggle with is how often they should be experiencing physical intimacy. The quick answer is probably more in the beginning of your relationship and then a little less as time goes on.

Typically, men desire physical intimacy more often than women, though this is not always the case.[3] Both men and women need to remember the importance of heart motive, though—why you are (or are not) desiring to engage in sex and whose needs you are putting first. Husbands and wives need to ask themselves these questions and consider what Paul says in 1 Corinthians 7

---

3. It may be helpful to clarify that there are at least two pathways to arousal: One is spontaneous and often begins internally, while the other is developed through external stimuli such as physical touch or emotional connection. Once generated, the desire may be equally strong. However, with any couple, it is not uncommon for each partner to have a different dominant form of origin for arousal. In a healthy, maturing relationship, both partners will recognize and accept this difference.

about the rights and obligations each spouse has toward the other regarding sexual intimacy. According to Scripture, abstaining from sexual intimacy should occur only with mutual consent and for the express purpose of prayer. Spouses should never treat sex as a reward to be earned or given. That said, we need to be aware of certain factors that will influence sexual desire.

First, sex reflects everything else going on in your life. You can't have a good sex life if you don't have a good relationship with each other. If you are frustrated with your spouse or stressed for any reason, the physical demonstrations of your love will obviously be less frequent. So, if you are experiencing disappointment in your physical relationship, think of it as a symptom of a greater disease and go looking for that illness. If you solve it, chances are good that your physical relationship will be repaired quite naturally.

Sexual desire can also be affected by physiological factors, such as the monthly fluctuations of a woman's hormones, certain prescription drugs, or a man's testosterone levels. Medications, including those prescribed for psychological issues, can have a significant effect on both sexual desire and performance. Both spouses need to be aware of such effects and continue to maintain an overall attitude of servanthood toward each other, offering, in a spirit of love, to suppress or jump-start their desires for the benefit of their spouse.

Sexual desire can also be affected by experience. Though sex may seem like "the most natural thing in the world," that doesn't mean it's automatically easy and enjoyable for everyone. You may benefit from some education and instruction. A friend of mine who is also a trained counselor shared an analogy that I thought was helpful. She pointed out that while breastfeeding is "natural," many women benefit from others' tips on how to help it feel more natural and be an experience of bonding with the baby. She went on to point out that this can also be the case with sex, as it is a skill that can be learned and improved on, leading to more satisfaction for both spouses.

Finally, we come to the question "What is permissible in the marriage bed?" As with all our other considerations, the issue here is one of the heart. Sexual intercourse is an intimate and vulnerable experience; this is the closest anyone will get to you, so what are they doing while they are there? If someone is selfish in this moment, it will create problems that radiate outward into the rest of your marriage.

The following questions may help you determine whether something is right for you:

- Does something trouble either your conscience or your spouse's? If one of you feels uneasy about doing something, immediately decide not to do it. A spouse should never encourage their partner to go against their biblically informed conscience. While our convictions can shift over time, this should happen individually and not because a spouse was pressured into submission. A spouse should feel safe and valued at all times—before, during, and after intimacy.

- Is the act under consideration an act of a servant or of a conqueror? Consider these words from Tim Challies, a pastor and the author of *Sexual Detox: A Guide for Guys Who Are Sick of Porn*, a book for those recovering from an addiction to pornography:

You know full well that many of the acts within pornography are acts of conquest, not acts of love and service. You know that in pornography the pleasure of the man is generally far greater and far more genuine than that of the woman. Do not subject your wife to acts that would make her feel like the mere means to an end, that would make her feel like she has been conquered instead of loved and nurtured, like she has been defiled instead of treasured.[4]

Using Challies's input, we can ask the following questions to evaluate any sexual act:

◊ Will the act be mutually enjoyable?
◊ Is my motive to serve my partner?
◊ Why do I want to do it?
◊ Bottom line: Can I thank God for it?

After assessing these questions, you may want to read Song of Solomon together, and you may be surprised by the intimate acts described in this book of the Bible. Yes, the book illustrates Christ's love for the church, but it also offers a candid discussion of love, and acts of love, between a man and a woman.

Ultimately, we must remember that sexual intimacy, like much of God's creation, is a wonderful, exciting, and pleasurable blessing when used as our Creator intended.

---

4. Tim Challies, "Sexual Detox IV: Detoxification," *Challies*, October 29, 2009, http://www.challies.com/christian-living/sexual-detox-iv-detoxification.

This means engaging in it with the right person (your spouse), at the right time (after marriage), and with the right motives (to produce children and/or enjoy each other). If we attempt to use this heavenly gift in any other way, it may still function to a degree during a season of passing pleasure. But sooner or later, we will encounter a problem and eventually face the judgment of God.

We must strive to remember that marriage is about service, not sex. If we wish to love God with all our heart, soul, mind, and strength, as well as love our spouse as ourselves, we will discover that our deepest desires, including our sexual desires, can be fulfilled in the most complete and extraordinary ways.

What About Birth Control?

When it comes to the issue of birth control, the first thing we need to remember is that technology is generally neutral; it is the *application* of technology that can be deemed good or bad.

Technically, we can discuss "birth control" from a preventative aspect or from a promotional aspect (using "controls" to increase the likelihood of pregnancy). Today's technologies enable us to do both. Therefore, before we ask if it is OK to use birth control, we must again ask, "What is sex for?"

If the only purpose of intercourse is to produce a child, then preventative forms of birth control must be ruled out. In this scenario, we should strongly consider the application of knowledge and techniques that increase the likelihood of conception. If done correctly, a couple could reduce the frequency of intercourse to just a few days each menstrual cycle when the woman is most fertile and then avoid intimacy for the rest of the month.[5] Additionally, if the only purpose of intercourse is to produce children, the couple should either time their honeymoon to coincide with the woman's peak ovulation or delay consummating their marriage until that time arrives.

This "procreation only" view implies that women who have undergone menopause, as well as couples in which one or both spouses are infertile, should refrain from sexual intercourse altogether. If the only purpose of intercourse is to produce children, then these couples should be entirely abstinent due to their inability to conceive.

Now, I've never met a person with such a severe view on the matter; they may exist, but this view seems to be the logical conclusion when you take a "procreation only" stance.

There are dangers on the opposite end of the spectrum as well. Those who want to prevent pregnancy "for a while" can become too caught up in pursuing their own pleasures before choosing the difficulties and sacrifices involved in parenting. Many young couples postpone having children because they are busy "enjoying themselves." The longer they delay, the easier it becomes to continue doing so. Suddenly, their twenties are gone or nearly gone, and they start thinking, "Wow, I guess it's time for us to consider having kids." At this point, it can be harder, though not impossible, for a woman to conceive, so those who know they want children should

---

5. This would actually be the inverse of the "calendar" method of birth control discussed later in the "Birth Control Technologies and Methods" section.

be actively considering how long is too long to delay. For most couples, the timing will not feel "perfect" and will require sacrifice and faith, so pray for God's will to be done in His timing.

Additionally, there is another category of couples to consider here: those who do not intend to have children at all. This may be because they fear the world into which the children would enter, because they worry about their financial ability to provide for them, because they feel unable to care for them while pursuing their own careers, or even because they're not sure they want to be parents. I would counsel these couples to reconsider God's basic command in Genesis 1:28: "God blessed them" and said, "Be fruitful and multiply." You may have very real and sincere concerns about parenting, but do you also trust God's ability to enable you to do whatever He calls you to do? I would encourage you to speak with your pastor, a trusted church leader, or others in the church about their experience with parenting, what their concerns were, and how God came through for them. Consider the blessings that God might want to pour out on you! God has commanded us to have children (Genesis 1:28) and tells us that they are a gift and a blessing from Him (Psalm 127:3–5).

Has God Condemned Birth Control?

Obviously, the first question we want to ask when considering any option is whether or not God has forbidden it. Regarding birth control, the answer is no; God has not forbidden it. Nowhere does the Bible say anything close to "You shall not prevent conception."

However, there is one important passage of Scripture for us to consider in light of this subject. This passage tells the story of Onan in Genesis:

> Then Judah took a wife for Er his firstborn, and her name was Tamar. But Er, Judah's firstborn, was wicked in the sight of the LORD, and the LORD killed him. And Judah said to Onan, "Go in to your brother's wife and marry her, and raise up an heir to your brother." But Onan knew that the heir would not be his; and it came to pass, when he went in to his brother's wife, that he emitted on the ground, lest he should give an heir to his brother. And the thing which he did displeased the LORD; therefore He killed him also. (Genesis 38:6–10)

Was Onan's attempt at birth control wrong? Yes, it was wrong, but that was because of his motives, not his method. Onan was selfish and did not want to take on the responsibility of providing for his brother's widow or raising a son to receive his older brother's inheritance. Without an heir, Onan would receive his brother's inheritance. The overwhelming opinion among commentators on this passage is that it focuses on Onan's motives rather than the method he employed.

The lesson we should learn from Onan is to examine our own motives. Why do we want to prevent or delay conception? If our motives are pure and not selfish (e.g., we want to wait until we graduate or until after a year-long, overseas deployment), it may be permissible to use various technologies or methods to assist us in doing so. You should discuss your thoughts on birth control as a couple, evaluate the facts regarding how various birth control methods function, and then make a thoughtful decision based on your own convictions.

Birth Control Technologies and Methods

Birth control can be classified into two categories: assisted and unassisted. Here, we will discuss some of the more common forms, how they operate, and whether they raise ethical concerns for Christians. Note that couples should make their decisions based on their own conscience. Just because a particular birth control method does not pose an ethical issue does not mean all couples will feel comfortable using it. Additionally, couples should investigate the efficacy rate for each method when used appropriately, as these rates will vary.

Unassisted Methods

- **Abstinence:** Obviously, never coming together sexually will prevent you from having children. However, Paul's instruction in 1 Corinthians 7 seems to override the option of abstinence, "except with consent for a time, that you may give yourselves to fasting and prayer" (v. 5).

- **Fertility Awareness Methods:** This approach involves scheduled abstinence and raises no ethical concerns. A woman is most fertile for a brief period of time within each monthly cycle. Couples can abstain from intercourse during this period of heightened fertility by using the calendar method or other indicators, such as basal body temperature, cervical fluid, cervical position, and various other bodily signs to track ovulation.

- **Withdrawal:** This prevents a viable sperm from contacting a viable egg and poses no ethical concerns. This method may not be as effective if applied inconsistently.

Assisted Methods

It is *critically* important for couples considering the following methods to exercise caution when discussing them with their health care provider. It is vital for you and your provider to share the same definitions of terms like *pregnancy* and *conception*. For instance, they may hold that life doesn't occur until a viable egg is implanted in the uterus and therefore may recommend a method that prohibits implantation. However, as Christians, we believe that life begins at conception and that any fertilized egg should have the opportunity to continue its development and attach to the uterine wall without impediment.

- **Barrier Methods:** These methods primarily include condoms, along with diaphragms, cervical caps, and spermicides like foams, creams, sponges, and vaginal suppositories. Barrier methods prevent viable sperm from reaching a viable egg and typically raise no ethical concerns.

- **Surgical Methods:** Surgical interventions, such as a male having a vasectomy or a woman having her "tubes tied," are, essentially, a more permanent version of a barrier method. In each case, sperm are prevented from reaching the egg. Fertilization and pregnancy are prevented. It is technically possible to reverse each procedure, but reversal is costly, complex, and not guaranteed. Surgical intervention does not pose a significant ethical concern. However, couples should give deep consideration to at least two questions. First, will their desire for any future children ever change? (E.g., what if the husband or wife were to pass away, and the remaining partner remarried, or what if one of their living children were to pass away?) Second, do they feel it is permissible to alter the function of the body as it was originally designed?

- **Chemical/Hormonal Contraception:** Contraception may include hormonal methods, such as birth control pills, patches, inserts, implants, and injections. Hormonal birth control is an unsettled issue for Christian ethicists and requires special care and concern from Christian couples. All forms of hormonally based chemical contraception (whether a combination of estrogen and progestin or progestin only) inhibit the endometrium (the lining of the uterus), preventing the implantation of a fertilized egg, if fertilization occurs. If we recognize life as beginning at the moment a viable sperm fertilizes a viable egg, then this method prevents that life from attaching to the uterus, where it would begin to grow. Consider the following excerpt from the official position statement on the issue from the Christian Medical & Dental Associations (CMDA):

  > Because this issue cannot be resolved with our current understanding, CMDA calls

upon researchers to further investigate the mechanisms of action of hormonal birth control. Additionally, because the possibility of abortive effects cannot be ruled out, prescribers of hormonal birth control should consider informing patients of this potential factor.[6]

There is a small chance of an egg being fertilized in a woman who is taking an oral contraceptive, but a chance does remain, and, if it were to occur, that viable egg would be denied the chance to implant in the uterus and continue developing as a human being. Therefore, couples will want to examine this issue seriously and in depth before choosing to use any form of hormonally based chemical contraception.[7]

- **Prohibitive or Flushing Methods:** These methods include any intrauterine device/system (IUD/IUS) and a chemical abortion pill, known as RU-486 or the "morning-after pill." Both work by creating an unsuitable environment in the uterus for a fertilized egg to implant. IUDs are also offered as a form of emergency contraception and have been shown to be capable of terminating a pregnancy when in-

---

6. "Christian Medical & Dental Association Position Statement," Eternal Perspective Ministries, March 13, 2010, https://www.epm.org/resources/2010/Mar/13/christian-medical-dental-association-position-stat/.

7. For additional reading on this subject, with well-documented footnotes, consult Andreas J. Köstenberger and David W. Jones, *God, Marriage, and Family: Rebuilding the Biblical Foundation*, 2nd ed. (Crossway, 2010), chap. 7 ("To Have or Not to Have Children").

serted up to five days after unprotected intercourse. A fertilized egg is an otherwise viable human life that could be sustained, could grow, and could thrive if allowed to implant. Robbing an otherwise viable life of the necessary opportunity to grow is ethically unacceptable for a Christian couple.

- **Abortion:** Whether through surgical or chemical means, abortion is the termination of a human life that has begun at conception. This is done by forcing an interruption in its natural development. Terminating the natural development of a viable life is ethically unacceptable for a Christian.

The choice to use birth control and the question of which methods to use represent significant decisions that should be made only after taking the time to educate yourselves, pray, and reach a consensus. The ethically appropriate option you choose may differ from those of other Christians, and that's perfectly OK. You must make decisions you are comfortable with so that you can stand with a clear conscience before God.

Summary

The core message of the Christian faith is that there is a God who created all of us and everything we see. He designed a world that would bring us purpose and pleasure as we love, serve, and worship Him. However, beginning with Adam and Eve, we have rebelled against our Creator, taking our lives and the resources He has given us and using them for our own enjoyment and purposes instead of as He intended. The result has been dysfunction, death, disease, and disaster on earth, culminating in His judgment throughout eternity. Fortunately, God is willing to forgive us for this rebellion and restore us to our original purposes and joy if we will simply submit to Him and receive the covering He offers us in Jesus Christ.

When we look at the issue of sex, we must view it through this lens. We will always be tempted to use this gift from God in our own ways, and if we do, we will face problems in our lives and judgment from Him. However, if we submit to Him and use sex as He intended, we will be blessed and fully able to enjoy sexual intimacy, free from shame or consequence.

In other words, every issue related to sex can be viewed as a matter of loyalty: Whom am I trying to please and obey in this realm—myself, my partner, or God? Who determines what is right and wrong, permitted and forbidden?

The answer, of course, must be God. He is the creator, designer, and giver of sex. To use it best, we should follow His original design, which is for one man to share this experience with the one woman to whom he is joined, till death parts them.

If we are to live up to this standard, we must avoid certain dangerous and powerful temptations. Fortunately, God promises to provide the strength we need to confront those challenges, and He offers us His forgiveness for the times we stumble. He promises to give us everything we need to live under His authority instead of living under the tyranny of our own attractions.

Reflection Questions – Chapter 3

1. What areas of your life might reflect an unhealthy "appetite" for things that don't align with God's design? How can you begin to retrain your desires with God's help?

2. Joel 2:25 speaks of God restoring what was lost. If you carry guilt or pain from past sexual sins — whether by choice or through being wronged — how might you invite God to restore your heart and renew your perspective?

3. Reflect on Matthew 5:27–28. In this passage, Jesus equates lust with adultery in the heart. What steps can you take to guard your heart and eyes from wandering thoughts or desires that dishonor God or others?

4. In 1 Corinthians 10:13, we read that God will provide us a way of escape from temptation. Can you recall a time when you faced temptation and found strength in God's provision? How can you rely on Him more intentionally in the future?

5. Dating couples should establish clear boundaries, such as not doing anything in private that they wouldn't do in public. Why do you think boundaries are so important for honoring God in relationships? List some practical ways couples can set and maintain these boundaries.

6. It is important to examine our motives and seek God's guidance when considering birth control. If applicable, discuss as a couple how you can ap-

proach this decision prayerfully, ensuring your choices align with your convictions.

7. As 1 Corinthians 7:3–5 highlights, spouses have the mutual responsibility to meet each other's needs. How can you and your spouse cultivate an attitude of servanthood in your physical relationship, especially during seasons in which intimacy might be challenging?

8. In 1 Timothy 5:1–2, we are instructed to treat others with purity, as family members. Whether you're single or married, how can you apply this principle in your interactions with the opposite sex to reflect God's heart for purity?

9. Proverbs 5:15–20 paints a vivid picture of finding delight in your spouse alone. How does this passage inspire you to view sexual intimacy as a gift from God? What steps can you take to align your desires with His design?

10. This chapter lists praying, reflecting on triggers, engaging in intimacy, and defending one's own heart as practical steps spouses can take to help themselves and each other overcome temptation. Which of these steps resonates most with you, and how can you implement it to overcome temptation in your life?

11. Because sex is a matter of loyalty to God over our attractions (in other words, authority over attraction), how can you cultivate a heart that seeks to please God above all else in your relationships and decisions about sexuality?

4

The Pitfall of Pornography

One of the most pervasive and pernicious forms of sexual sin in our day is rarely addressed from Christian pulpits or in Bible studies. Pornography ensnares both men and women, teenagers and adults, Christians and non-Christians. It destroys marriages and ruins lives. While sex is a good and beautiful gift created to unite husband and wife in deeper intimacy, pornography twists the focus of sex inward, causing those who engage in it to become more selfish and isolated.

An analysis of internet traffic in the United States from September to November 2023 shows that three of the top twenty most visited sites on the internet were porn sites. One of them gets twice as much traffic as Instagram, two of them beat ESPN.com, and all three of them get more clicks than the Fox News home page.[1]

---

1. Tiago Bianchi, "Leading Websites in the United States from September to November 2023, by Total Visits," Statista, March 14, 2024, https://www.statista.com/statistics/1456422/most-visited-websites-total-visits-united-states/.

When you consider worldwide internet traffic, in November 2023, the top three most popular websites in the world were predictably Google, YouTube, and Facebook. But the next two? Porn sites. Two of the top five most popular websites in the entire world serve up a corrupted version of sex, ensnaring millions. Four of the fifteen most popular websites globally are porn sites that collectively generate more than 30 billion monthly visits.[2]

These statistics are depressing but not shocking. People have always been drawn to sexual sin. The word *pornography* itself comes from ancient Greek. *Pornē* means "prostitute," and *graphe* means "to write." So pornography "was originally defined as any work of art or literature depicting the life of prostitutes."[3] A variant of that word, *pornēa* (referring to "sexual immorality"), is used throughout the New Testament. I share this so you know two things.

First, pornography, like all sexual sin, has been around for a very long time. When God first relayed His Ten Commandments to Moses on Mount Sinai, He forbade man to covet his neighbor's wife (Exodus 20:17) and also commanded him not to commit adultery (Exodus 20:14) — sex with someone who is not your spouse. Don't miss the fact that these commands were specifically given to *God's own people*. In other words, even people

---

2. Tiago Bianchi, "Most Popular Websites Worldwide as of November 2023, by Total Visits," Statista, last updated May 21, 2025, https://www.statista.com/statistics/1456422/most-visited-websites-total-visits-united-states/.

3. John Philip Jenkins, "pornography," *Encyclopaedia Britannica*, last updated December 20, 2024, https://www.britannica.com/topic/pornography.

who know God need to be told, "Keep your eyes and your desires under control."

The second reason I mention the origin of the word *pornography* is this: It helps us remember that it's more than just pictures or videos. Pornography has always included writing. Even if there are no images, pornographic writing or explicit descriptions (e.g., in novels) can be a source of stumbling—particularly for women. Traditional romance novels and more modern adaptations like the *Fifty Shades of Grey* series have specifically targeted female readers, luring them to covet what they don't have or don't experience and to be dissatisfied with their current circumstances. Steamy sex scenes are embedded in a "compelling" plot, and readers rationalize their indulgence because "it's all just part of the story." The *Encyclopaedia Britannica* defines *pornography* as a "representation of sexual behaviour in books, pictures, statues, films, and other media that is intended to cause sexual excitement."[4]

Pay close attention to the last part of that definition. While pornography can be presented in many different forms of media, it always has the same purpose: It is *intended* to arouse. That is why we are so drawn to it; it is also why we are quick to defend ourselves when other believers question us about it.

The Game of Justifications

In 1964, the US Supreme Court was hearing arguments in a case regarding the nature of obscenity and pornography. Justice Potter Stewart was asked to define hard-

---

4. Jenkins, "pornography."

core pornography and famously responded, "I know it when I see it." (Ironically, he made this statement in his justification that he didn't think a sexually explicit film technically violated obscenity laws.)[5]

If pornographic material is created with the intention to arouse, we need to be honest enough to admit that we know it when we see it (or when we read it or hear it). Yet we are often tempted to justify our actions to others, to ourselves, and even to God.

Be honest: Do you find yourself rationalizing reading books with sexual content or watching TV shows or movies that regularly use sexual language or imagery? When these things come up in conversation with other believers, do you try to explain away or justify material that sexually excites you? For example,

- "Oh, this book I like isn't *really* pornography. I'm not one of 'those people.' I just really like the story, even if it happens to include a few sex scenes."

- "This new show has good acting, fascinating storylines, and amazing scenery. It may have some nudity, but it's not the same thing as *porn*."

- "These are just videos on YouTube or Instagram. Maybe the people on screen are dressed a bit provocatively, but they still have clothes on, and they are not doing anything sexual."

- "Look, I just really like this song and the way it sounds. I don't focus on the lyrics."

---

5. Wikipedia, "I Know It When I See It," last modified January 22, 2025, 14:35 (UTC), https://en.wikipedia.org/wiki/I_know_it_when_I_see_it.

The Pitfall of Pornography

My friend, could you stand before God and say sincerely that such things do not cause you to be sexually excited? You may be able to tell yourself or others that "it's not porn." But does it have a pornographic *effect* on you? Is that novel or program or social media content "intended to cause sexual excitement"? Does it lead your heart to places that God says you should not go?

Consider the words of Job, written more than three thousand years ago. He says:

> I have made a covenant with my eyes; why then should I look upon a young woman? For what is the allotment of God from above, and the inheritance of the Almighty from on high? Is it not destruction for the wicked, and disaster for the workers of iniquity? Does He not see my ways, and count all my steps? (Job 31:1–4)

Job essentially says, "If I give in to this attraction, this lust, God sees and knows and judges." Friend, God has an opinion about whom and what you're attracted to. This is why our goal is to submit our sexuality to the authority of Jesus. We say, "God, You get to tell me how and when to use my sexuality and to whom and what I should be attracted."

Attraction can be a normal and positive thing when it is under God's authority! Ideally, it's part of how you meet your spouse. But when your attraction is driven by your fleshly desires and is not submitted to God's authority, it will pull you into things you have no purpose being a part of. That's when you need to make a covenant like Job to shift your eyes and your attention away from "uncleanness" (Colossians 3:5). You need to escape the moment of temptation (even physically) and tell yourself, "That's not for me." If you give in to curiosity or desire, it can lead you to things you'll be ashamed of, things you'll regret, and things that may destroy you and your ability to form healthy relationships.

Your sexuality is a powerful thing. It should be a magnetic force at the center of your marriage propelling you toward your spouse. But, left ungoverned, it can also be the destructive energy of a life given over to suppressing the truth and pursuing the self. The things that seem to excite you can actually destroy you.

Let me show you what I mean.

An Appetite for Destruction

If we are going to be successful in our fight against the temptation of pornography, we need to understand exactly how destructive and diabolical it is.

First, *pornography damages your relationship with God.* Pornography—in all its forms and formats—is a distortion, a twisting of what God in His goodness designed and gave to humanity. It says to God, "I know what You gave, and it's not enough." It says, "I want something else" or "I want more." It tells God, "You don't know what You're doing. You don't know what's best. I do. I like this."

This is the exact ploy that Satan used in the Garden of Eden. He convinced Adam and Eve to be discontent with the good and satisfying gifts that God had richly provided. The serpent enticed them to covet the one thing that God had drawn a clear boundary around. They believed Satan's lie that God was denying their greatest need, so they chose to take what was not theirs. In the millennia since that first temptation, the game has remained the same: We are tempted to doubt that God's good provision and gracious boundaries are for our good, and we transgress because we believe we know better. We suppress the truth we have been given, choosing to believe the promise of the lie.

Second, *pornography destroys your relationships with others*. It reduces your likelihood of finding satisfaction in your spouse. As a pastor, I've come across this many times in counseling—situations in which the person using pornography eventually finds themselves less and less interested in their spouse. It becomes more and more difficult for them to be satisfied in their "normal" relationship. This makes sense because, in a way, pornography is just marketing: It entices you to want what you do not have by convincing you that you deserve it and cannot live without it. It presents sexual experiences as normal, something that other people enjoy all the time but that you're missing out on.

Then you look at your spouse, and you're disappointed. You may not admit it, but you think, "Why aren't you like that?" or "Why can't we do that?"

This dissatisfaction may occur in terms of physical comparison, but it can also apply to emotional connections just as easily. If you are consuming pornography that presents a wildly romantic and exciting affair, only to look up and feel bored because you and your spouse are no longer in the "honeymoon phase" of your relationship, you may fall into discontentment, wondering why your relationship or experience is not like the pornographic one.

Comparison is the thief of joy.

Authority over Attraction

When you stock your mind with romantic or arousing images and ideas that don't involve your actual spouse, you're stacking the deck against them by setting an unrealistic standard. At the same time, you are also making it harder and harder to appreciate and enjoy the relationships you have because you keep thinking about the ones you don't.

If you are a single person, it is even more important that you avoid the illusion of pornography. While you might be tempted to look to erotic novels or sexual images as a substitute for the real thing, you are only setting yourself up to reject a real relationship when it happens. When you have trained your mind and arousal to be attracted to the lies that pornography peddles, real human companionship will always fall short. Romantic relationships can be challenging, even if both people are believers, because we are all sinners in need of grace from God and each other. Pornography presents a thin facsimile of love that demands nothing of us and serves only our selfish interests. But this was never part of God's design for human sexuality.

Single people who consume pornography are training their minds and hearts to expect a kind of relationship that was never intended for them. And, as a pastor, I can't tell you the number of times I have heard someone say, "I thought getting married would fix this for me, but it didn't." Similarly, I don't know that I've ever heard someone say, "Marriage solved all my problems with pornography and lust."

Finally, *pornography will inevitably dehumanize you*. Rather than being in control of your desires and emotions, you will become driven by them like an animal, reduced to nothing more than your interests and impulses. You will begin to regard other people as mere shapes and appearances, thinking of them only in terms of their ability to satisfy your infinite appetite. This is a dangerous situation to be in because your sexual appetite is never completely satisfied when left to its own devices. Instead, it begins to curve toward escalation. Like any addiction, you will require more or different stimuli to reach new levels of excitement. Recent studies have shown that repeated use of pornography actually damages people neurologically.[6] For those who have already started down the road of pornography use, apart from God healing you with an instantaneous miracle (which is possible), it will take time to break the addiction and rewire your mind.

When you engage in pornography use, you trade away your freedom for another hit of satisfaction. While you may begin by simply being curious about something, you quickly become controlled by it and, eventually, chained to it. For some, the path becomes darker, deeper, and more twisted as it pursues something new and fresh. Your appetite ultimately trains you to desire what is evil and unlawful. No one starts with the most hardcore or depraved elements of por-

---

6. See Dr. Joe Malone, host, *The Pregnancy Help Podcast*, "Women's Sexual Wellness," February 12, 2024, https://pregnancyhelp.blubrry.net/2024/02/12/womens-sexual-wellness-dr-joe-malone/. For additional published research, see Donald L. Hilton and Clark Watts, "Pornography Addiction: A Neuroscience Perspective," *Surgical Neurology International* 2 (February 2011): 19, https://doi.org/10.4103/2152-7806.76772. See also Simone Kühn and Jürgen Gallinat, "Brain Structure and Functional Connectivity Associated with Pornography Consumption: The Brain on Porn," *JAMA Psychiatry* 71, no. 7 (2014): 827–834, https://doi.org/10.1001/jamapsychiatry.2014.93.

nography; rather, you work your way there by slowly expanding your boundaries.

For some, it takes waking up to the reality that they have reached a level of sexual degradation they never expected. Just as Paul describes in Romans 1, sexual sin devolves into darker and more unnatural desires. There are many accounts of men convicted and sentenced for heinous sexual crimes who report a history of pornography use. The desire for greater arousal and new thrills led them to pursue sexual experiences they never would have considered acceptable before. Sexual sin deceives us, degrades us, and destroys us—one decision at a time.

The USA Gymnastics Olympics team was rocked with scandal a few years ago when it came out that Larry Nassar, the team doctor, had been sexually abusing female athletes. Investigations revealed he had molested more than 250 women. During his trial, Rachael Denhollander, a Christian woman who was one of the abuse survivors, took the stand and told him,

> You have become a man ruled by selfish and perverted desires, a man defined by his daily choices repeatedly to feed that selfishness and perversion. You chose to pursue your wickedness no matter what it cost others, and the opposite of what you have done is for me to choose to love sacrificially, no matter what it costs me.[7]

---

7. Quoted in Drew Dyck, *Your Future Self Will Thank You: Secrets to Self-Control from the Bible & Brain Science* (Moody Publishers, 2019), 30. See also People v. Nassar, 974 N.W. 2d 833 (2018).

The Pitfall of Pornography

Notice two starkly different things there: first, the ability to forgive at great personal cost by someone who has received the love of Christ, and second, the condemnation that Nassar had *become* this monster by making *daily* choices to feed his selfishness. No one starts at this level of wickedness. But the trail can lead you there. If you know that, why would you follow it?

In 2023, I listened to a podcast with Jason Portnoy, who started his career at PayPal in the early days with men like Peter Thiel. Portnoy then became the first chief financial officer at Palantir Technologies. He was a Silicon Valley unicorn with skyrocketing wealth. He also had a growing addiction to pornography that led him into self-destructive behaviors. He began by looking at pictures, moved on to videos, and then eventually used Craigslist to find hookups and escort services.

Even though Portnoy is not a follower of Jesus, he was able (by God's common grace) to realize the destructiveness of pornography in his life. In the interview, he said,

> What I do think is very bad is porn in any amount at any time. I think that zero is the right amount. I think it is toxic. I think it is hurting our young men. . . . I think it is hurting young women. I think it's just bad, just all around.[8]

---

8. Tim Ferriss, host, *The Tim Ferriss Show*, podcast, episode 600, "Jason Portnoy of PayPal, Palantir, and More—Porn Addiction, the Corrosiveness of Secrets, Healing Wounds, Escaping Shame Cycles, and Books to Change Your Life," June 15, 2022, https://tim.blog/2022/06/15/jason-portnoy/.

All these terrible consequences do not even take into account the countless lives that have been destroyed within the pornography industry itself. The people behind the images on your screen are all image-bearers of God who have chosen darkness and become enslaved by it themselves. There are also men and women who were forced into a life of sexual degradation through the wicked actions of others and who could not see a way of escape. There are hundreds of stories online detailing drug abuse, sexual violence, personal trauma, and self-harm that are hidden behind the arousing images you consume. Pornography damages the lives of both the image-bearers who create it and those who consume it.

If pornography is your personal struggle, you may have been sold the lie that it's a personal choice that doesn't hurt anyone else. The reality is that pornography of all kinds has destructive consequences:

- It damages your relationship with God through its inherent denial that He is sufficient to meet your needs. Each sinful choice keeps you from pursuing Him with your whole heart.

- Porn hampers or undercuts your real relationships with the opposite sex in general and with your (current or potential) spouse in particular.

- It dehumanizes you by making you a slave to your cravings, desiring more and more stimulation at greater costs.

- And, ultimately, pornography steals you away from the people in your life who need you. You can become less engaged with your spouse and detached with your kids. If you are caught in your sin

The Pitfall of Pornography

by your family, it could lead to feelings of betrayal that may take years to heal.

Pornography wrecks marriages and destroys homes. If you choose to embrace darkness instead of walking in light, you will isolate yourself from the people around you in your home, church, and community who want to love you, grow with you, and hold you accountable.

This is not God's plan for you, nor is it why He made you. You're supposed to be making the lives of others better for His glory, and they're supposed to do the same for you. And no matter how long you have been trapped in pornography addiction, He can still free you from it, if you will repent and come to Him for cleansing and rescue. It can happen. It will happen. But it starts by submitting your sexuality to Jesus instead of allowing it to rule over you.

This is why Jesus was so severe when He dealt with sexual sin. Think of what He said in His famous Sermon on the Mount:

> You have heard that it was said to those of old, "You shall not commit adultery." But I say to you that whoever looks at a woman to lust for her has already committed adultery with her in his heart. If your right eye causes you to sin, pluck it out and cast it from you; for it is more profitable for you that one of your members perish, than for your whole body to be cast into hell. And if your right hand causes you to sin, cut it off and cast it from you; for it is more profitable for you that one of your members perish, than for your whole body to be cast into hell. (Matthew 5:27–30)

Jesus is being emphatic here, exaggerating to make a point. But rather than writing His statement off as overkill, let's not miss what He is getting at: Jesus wants us to take desire and sexual sin seriously—*in all their forms.* Remember the analogy of the fireplace? If you keep the fire of intimacy within the fireplace of marriage, all is well. If you move the fire into another part of the house, the whole thing burns down. Jesus is telling us not to play with sexual sin, tolerate it, or ignore it. Instead, we are to root out and destroy sexual sin in our lives at all costs to escape self-destruction in this life and the next.

Escaping the Trap

So where do we go from here? In chapter 6, we will look at steps we can take to resist pornography and other temptations in a sex-soaked world. We will also examine how we can respond when sexual sin ensnares people we know and love. But before moving on, let's pause and review two important truths in our framework of pursuing holy sexuality.

First, remember that distinctions matter. If you have been engaging in pornography use (of any kind), this chapter may be provoking strong responses. That happens when light shines into the darkness, exposing what is hidden. But if you are a Christian, remember that there is a difference between *conviction* and *condemnation*. For the Christian, condemnation comes from the flesh and the Enemy, and its goal is to drive us away from God. Conviction comes from the Holy Spirit and drives us toward Jesus through repentance. That means it is right to "feel bad" about your sin, if it leads you to repentance. It is not OK if your bad feelings cause you to hide from the light and continue suppressing the truth. Consider how Paul carefully distinguishes between godly sorrow (genuine conviction of sin) and worldly sorrow (self-condemnation and fear of judgment) in 2 Corinthians 7:8–11:

> For even if I made you sorry with my letter, I do not regret it; though I did regret it. For I perceive that the same epistle made you sorry, though only for a while. Now I rejoice, not that you were made sorry, but that your sorrow led to repentance. For you were made sorry in a godly manner, that you might suffer loss from us in nothing. For godly sorrow produces repentance leading to salvation, not to be regretted; but the sorrow of the world produces death. For observe this very thing, that you sorrowed in a godly manner: What diligence it produced in you, what clearing of yourselves, what indignation, what fear, what vehement desire, what zeal, what vindication! In all things you proved yourselves to be clear in this matter.

Godly sorrow leads not to self-condemnation but to active and eager repentance.

It is also essential for you to understand the difference between *temptation* and *sin*. Jesus was "in all points tempted as we are, yet without sin" (Hebrews 4:15). In the same way, you can be tempted sexually without being guilty of sin from the temptation itself. Sin occurs when we are "drawn away by [our] own desires and enticed" (James 1:14). That's why we are instructed to "flee sexual immorality" (1 Corinthians 6:18). We must resist all forms of sexual temptation to avoid falling into the snare of sin.

This distinction between temptation and sin is important. You will continue to be tempted sexually, especially if this has been an area of struggle for you in the past. As you keep fighting the good fight against lust every day, the Enemy will tempt you and then try to condemn you for being tempted. Do not give in to condemnation. In your struggle against sexual sin, know that the hosts of heaven are on your side, cheering you on in your pursuit of holy sexuality.

The second truth is this: You can change. You may be discouraged because you have tried and failed to resist the siren call of pornography. You know that it is destroying you, and you want to obey God, but in moments of weakness you give in. You wonder if there is any point in fighting and failing. You are tempted to think you are just permanently stuck and broken. Maybe God can't really change your heart, or perhaps He doesn't really care enough to do so.

Friend, the answer to all these doubts, based on God's own testimony, is *do not give up*! It doesn't matter how long you have been enslaved to this sin; Christ came to proclaim freedom for the captives and healing for the brokenhearted (Luke 4:18). Your change might look like an overnight miracle, or it might look like a mud-soaked obstacle course. But listen to me: Just because it's hard doesn't mean you're doing it wrong.

In Romans 7, Paul writes about his own struggle with temptation and how he feels torn between the good that he desires to do and the sin that his flesh is drawn toward. In the end, he cries out, "O wretched man that I am! Who will deliver me from this body of death? I thank

God—through Jesus Christ our Lord! So then, with the mind I myself serve the law of God, but with the flesh the law of sin" (Romans 7:24–25). And what is the very next thing the apostle writes at the start of Romans 8?

> There is therefore now *no condemnation* to those who are in Christ Jesus, who do not walk according to the flesh, but according to the Spirit. For the law of the Spirit of life in Christ Jesus has *made me free* from the law of sin and death. (Romans 8:1–2, emphasis mine)

In other words, while we struggle and strain against sin and wage war against our flesh and its weakness, we do so in hope. Jesus Christ died and rose again to deliver us from the "body of death." Therefore, all who are in Christ Jesus are no longer condemned but are set free from the law of sin and death. Praise God for this promised deliverance!

That hope is how we wage war against sin without giving up. We know that God's will is for our sanctification (1 Thessalonians 4:3), so we fight on with the strength He provides. Facing and overcoming difficulty and struggle in our lives produces strength, and God wants you to be strong for yourself and for others. The same gospel that saves your soul will set you free from this sin. Listen to this promise of Scripture—one of my personal favorites:

> No temptation has overtaken you except such as is common to man; but God is faithful, who will not allow you to be tempted beyond what you are able, but with the temptation will also make

the way of escape, that you may be able to bear it. (1 Corinthians 10:13)

Sexual temptation does not have to defeat you, because your God is able to help you escape the trap. Change can happen. Victory over sin is possible in Jesus's name.

Jesus doesn't love you because you're good; He loves you because *He's* good. He wants to heal you, help you, and make you the man or woman He designed you to be in every area of life. Invite Him in and talk to Him about your sin. Ask for His help to flee temptation. Begin submitting your sexuality to Jesus today so that you can live a life that glorifies the God who made you.

Reflection Questions – Chapter 4

1. How can recognizing that God created sex and sexuality help shift our view of it from something shameful to something good and purposeful? How does this perspective affect your approach to sexual temptation and sin?

2. Discuss the ways in which pornography can damage one's relationship with God. What are some practical steps you can take to avoid or overcome the temptation to engage in pornography?

3. Pornography can negatively affect our relationships with others. How have you seen pornography impact relationships in your life or in the lives of those around you? How can one rebuild trust and intimacy after such damage?

4. Job made a covenant with his eyes to avoid looking at women with lust. How can this principle be applied in today's digital age in which images and media are ubiquitous? What specific actions can you take to uphold this covenant?

5. How can understanding the difference between temptation and sin affect your self-perception and spiritual growth? Share an example of a time when distinguishing between these two helped you in your walk with Christ.

6. Consider the difference we noted between conviction (which leads us to repentance) and condemnation (which drives us away from God). How can you differentiate between the two in your own life? How

can you ensure that conviction leads you toward positive change rather than discouragement?

7. Reflect on the promises from 1 Corinthians 10:13 about God providing a way of escape from temptation. How does this promise offer hope and encouragement for someone struggling with sexual sin? What are some practical ways to rely on God's help in overcoming these challenges?

5

Against Nature: Submitting Sinful Desire to God's Authority

Charles Spurgeon pastored a church in London more than 150 years ago. In his day, he was known internationally and was considered the most famous preacher of his generation. Transcripts of his sermons were regularly published, sold, and read around the world. Spurgeon said this about Romans 1 in a sermon he preached near the end of his ministry:

> [It is] a dreadful portion of the Word of God. I should hardly like to read it all through aloud; it is not intended to be so used. Read it at home, and be startled at the awful vices of the Gentile world.[1]

This statement seems ironic to me because Paul intended for his epistle to be read out loud to the church

---

1. Charles Haddon Spurgeon, "Inexcusable Irreverence and Ingratitude," The Spurgeon Center, accessed February 19, 2025, https://www.spurgeon.org/resource-library/ sermons/inexcusable-irreverence-and-ingratitude/#flipbook/.

in Rome. But Spurgeon lived at a time when the morality of the nation was different than that of the first century. In Spurgeon's time, there were no openly homosexual couples; there was no gay marriage and no pride month. You didn't even talk about these things in polite company.

The world has changed radically since then. Today, things look much like they did in the first century. Sins and vices that were common in ancient Rome are common once again, so the church needs to talk about them again. This means taking a clear-eyed look at what the Bible has to say about homosexual attraction and behavior.

As I wrote in the introduction, I am a pastor, not a professor, and I'm certainly not an expert on every detail of this subject. I'm also not a licensed counselor or therapist, so I might not speak with clarity or insight regarding your personal situation. I'm not a politician, nor am I advocating for or against any particular legislation. I'm an ambassador of the Kingdom of God, so my goal is to tell you what God has said about these things. I neither represent nor speak on behalf of anyone or anything else.

My goal in this chapter (and in the book as a whole) is to be both kind and clear—to help people love Jesus more and not to drive anyone away. I have no desire to be provocative. I'm not trying to go viral with a hot take on these issues. But the truth of Scripture is offensive to us when it challenges our self-rule.

You need to understand that God is both intolerant of sin and deeply merciful to repentant sinners. Jesus said harsh things about sexual sins and then died a harsh death for them. Because of Jesus's substitutionary sacrifice, all sin, including sexual sin, can be forgiven. You can be cleansed. There are fresh starts and new beginnings for everyone in Christ.

We will begin our exploration of this cultural, hot-button issue by reviewing the flow of Romans 1. As we have already seen, God reveals Himself to people all over the world, all throughout time. However, rather than worshipping Him, mankind, in its rebellion, suppresses the truth He reveals. Many people would rather live life their own way without being responsible to God. God graciously puts up with that for a while as He patiently calls people to Himself. But at some point, He gives stubborn rebels over to their selfish desires, which lead them in all kinds of destructive directions. This "giving over" is epitomized by sexual sin in general and homosexuality specifically:

> For this reason God gave them up to vile passions. For even their women exchanged the natural use for what is against nature. Likewise also the men, leaving the natural use of the woman, burned in their lust for one another, men with men committing what is shameful, and receiving in themselves the penalty of their error which was due. (Romans 1:26–27)

This is a harsh condemnation of homosexuality. It does not sit well with some of your neighbors, friends, or family members. It may not even sit well with you, as you read it. But do not miss the fact that this warning is addressed not only to present-day America. This is what God has *always* said in His Word. Society has changed, but God has not.

Why is God opposed to homosexuality? Because homosexuality rejects God's most fundamental design for humanity: He created man and woman to complement one another and to be fruitful and multiply.

Let's start by seeking to understand the prevalence of homosexuality in our culture.

How Big Is the Issue?

According to nearly all polling, it appears that Americans vastly overestimate the homosexual population in the United States, though a notable trend is occurring among the youngest generation:

- When Americans were polled in 2013 about what percentage of the population identified as homosexual, the average response was around 23 percent.[2] While it is difficult to be precise, the reality, according to most researchers, was around 3 to 4 percent of Americans at that time.[3]

- According to the United Kingdom's Office for National Statistics (a government agency), 1 per-

---

2. George Diepenbrock, "Majority Overestimates U.S. Gay Population, Could Influence Gay Rights Policies, Researchers Find," *KU News*, The University of Kansas, October 16, 2017, https://news.ku.edu/news/article/2017/10/12/majority-overestimates-us-gay-population-could-influence-gay-rights-policies-researchers.

3. "Share of Respondents Who Identified as Lesbian, Gay, Bisexual or Transgender in the United States from 2012 to 2023," Statista, accessed February 19, 2025, https://www.statista.com/statistics/719674/american-adults-who-identify-as-homosexual-bisexual-or-transgender/.

cent of people in England self-identified as gay in 2013.[4]

- A Gallup poll conducted in early 2024 found similar numbers for the United States: 1.4 percent of US adults identified as gay, and 1.2 percent identified as lesbian.[5] When combined with other nonheterosexual categories, that works out to about nine million LGBT[6] Americans.

- The numbers are radically higher among younger generations. About 15 percent of Gen Z (born between 1997 and 2012) identified as bisexual in 2024. That's roughly one out of every seven people between the ages of 13 and 27 in the United States. This is more common among young women than it is among young men. About 20 percent of Gen Z women identify as bisexual, as opposed to 6.9 percent of Gen Z men.[7]

There are at least two important ideas to take away from these statistics. First, we tend to overestimate

---

4. Mona Chalabi, "Gay Britain: What Do the Statistics Say?," *The Guardian*, October 3, 2013, https://www.theguardian.com/politics/reality-check/2013/oct/03/gay-britain-what-do-statistics-say. Note that, while this article is more than ten years old, the overall population numbers remain consistent with recent Gallup data for the United States.

5. Jeffrey M. Jones, "LGBTQ+ Identification in U.S. Now at 7.6%," Gallup, March 13, 2024, https://news.gallup.com/poll/611864/lgbtq-identification.aspx.

6. LGBTQ+ stands for "lesbian, gay, bisexual, transgender, queer, and other sexual identities."

7. Jones, "LGBTQ+ Identification."

how common these other forms of sexuality are among the general population. That's probably due to the combined support of media coverage and community allies. Representation of these alternative sexualities in pop culture tends to outpace actual representation in society. In addition, when you see a rainbow flag in your neighborhood, it might not be because that person is gay but because they are signaling their support of those who are. If you just go by what you *see*, the numbers may seem large, but if you go by what people *do*, the population is relatively small. Another takeaway here is that something has suddenly had a radical impact on young people, especially young girls, to cause such a shift in self-identity. We will come back to this shortly.

Contributing Factors

It is crucial to understand that homosexuality is not a uniform experience. There are multiple factors that may contribute to same-sex attraction. The person who identifies as homosexual may have experienced any or all of these factors. And, of course, there are also people who experience these factors but don't experience same-sex attraction at all.

Abuse

One key factor that may contribute to sexual confusion is having a personal history of abuse:

- Researchers at Vanderbilt University and Vanderbilt University Medical Center found that 83 percent of LGBQ individuals "reported going through adverse childhood experiences such as sexual and emotional abuse."[8]

- In another study of homosexual and bisexual men, 35.5 percent reported being sexually abused as children.[9]

- In yet another study, gay men and lesbian women reported a significantly higher rate of same-sex molestation as children than did heterosexual men and women. About 46 percent of the homosexual men reported being molested by another male, as compared to 7 percent of the heterosexual men surveyed who were also molested. About 22 percent of lesbian women reported being molested by another female as children, compared to 1 percent of heterosexual women surveyed who were also molested.[10]

---

8. Jake Lowary, "Study Finds LGBQ People Report Higher Rates of Adverse Childhood Experiences than Straight People, Worse Mental Health as Adults," *VUMC News*, Vanderbilt University Medical Center, February 24, 2022, https://news.vumc.org/2022/02/24/study-finds-lgbq-people-report-higher-rates-of-adverse-childhood-experiences-than-straight-people-worse-mental-health-as-adults/. The study discussed in this article (published February 23, 2022, in the *Journal of American Medical Association Psychiatry*) used data from a 2019 Centers for Disease Control and Prevention survey.

9. William R. Lenderking et al., "Childhood Sexual Abuse Among Homosexual Men," *Journal of General Internal Medicine* 12, no. 4 (1997): 250–253, https://doi.org/10.1046/j.1525-1497.1997.012004250.x.

10. Marie E. Tomeo et al., "Comparative Data of Childhood and Adolescence Molestation in Heterosexual and Homosexual Persons," *Archives of Sexual Behavior* 30 (October 2001): 535–541, https://doi.org/10.1023/a:1010243318426.

Let's be extremely clear: This is not true in every case. Not all homosexuals were abused as children, and not everyone who was abused as a child developed homosexual attraction. However, the research shows that there is a correlation between childhood abuse and same-sex attraction in adulthood.

That connection between abuse and broken sexuality should grieve us. All abuse should grieve us as a violation of God's Word and as an attack on someone made in God's image. Additionally, these connections should remind us that brokenness often breeds brokenness.

Addiction

A second factor that feeds same-sex attraction is addiction. We discussed this in the previous chapter about pornography. I have had multiple conversations with men who identified as heterosexual (some even married with children) but whose addiction to pornography drove them to explore homosexual content to find a new thrill. Addiction always drives people to seek something new, something more, because they have tried everything else.

When it comes to addiction, we should also recognize the role of drug use and its contribution to sexual encounters. Drug use lowers inhibitions and can make you more susceptible to temptation in ways you may not anticipate. In fact, men and women who have come out of the pornography industry and sex trade often report of extensive drug use by those involved in order to lower inhibitions and numb mental and psychological discomfort. The world of addiction is hard and ugly, often taking you to places you did not intend to go. The good news is that, with help, you can return to where you want to be.

Attention

The third factor contributing to same-sex attraction and embracing the LGBTQ+ identity grouping is a desire for attention. Until the 1960s, homosexuality was considered socially shameful and was kept out of view of the mainstream. However, that decade proved to be a definite turning point in American culture. Previously, we expected individuals to submit their desires or ambitions to the service of ideals and groups beyond themselves, such as the nuclear family, the church, and the community. This perspective shifted dramatically during the 1960s, though the seeds of this shift were planted in academia and the arts much earlier. Personal autonomy and expression were now being upheld as the greatest human good. Young people in particular were encouraged to shake off the chains of past generations and pursue individual freedom. The fallout from this has been felt over the last sixty years:

- As birth control became more readily available, sex was untethered from the risk of pregnancy, and sexual expression and exploration became more widespread.

- Science was presented as the usurper of religion, and Christian tradition and theology were denigrated and dismissed. Therefore, theological teaching about self and sexuality were likewise thrown out.

- Today, basic tenets of the so-called "hard" sciences like anatomy, biology, and physiology are being rewritten or ignored to conform to the new gender-fluidity dogma. "Softer" sciences like psychology and sociology are now considered more credible in describing sexual identity.

Today, the autonomous self is king, and all institutions (from the family to the church to the state itself) are told to bow down to the self-constructed identity of the individual.[11]

Because of these widespread cultural changes, nearly a century in the making, we live in a culture that not only tolerates or acknowledges LGBTQ+ identities but indeed celebrates them as brave expressions of personal autonomy. Those who declare their new, alternative identity are championed and seen as heroes. It should not be surprising that young girls who experience a special bond or closeness with other women start to confuse healthy friendship with same-sex attraction.

Imagine an adolescent girl who is constantly told on social media that it's cool to be LGBTQ+. She may decide that her affection for her female best friend and her desire to go with a boy to Homecoming must mean she is actually bisexual and not just a normal adolescent girl. Then, when she announces her newly embraced identity to her social media circle, she receives a flood of affirming messages from her peers, complete with the serotonin boost from the likes, shares, and comments that flood in. Additionally, she may get significantly more social clout and attention as a newly minted member of the LGBTQ+

---

11. For further information on the rise of the autonomous self in modern culture and a detailed review of how we got to this moment in history, see Carl R. Trueman's book *Strange New World: How Thinkers and Activists Redefined Identity and Sparked the Sexual Revolution* (Crossway, 2022).

community than she ever did as a boring, ordinary heterosexual girl. The ripple effect comes when the next girl, who watches this process happen, starts to wonder if she may like girls too.

Cultural forces press young people today (and young girls in particular) to embrace an identity that is driven more by confusion and a desire for social approval than by conviction and certainty. We need to teach younger generations (and model for them) that close same-sex friendships are a blessing and a gift. You can feel affection and loyalty to someone of the same sex without having any kind of sexual feelings toward them.[12]

Tim Keller once gave a helpful example of how shifting cultural standards can shape our self-perception.[13] He said to imagine being a Viking living about a thousand years ago. The pressure of your culture tells you to be adventurous and violent—conquering, pillaging, and destroying other villages. Your parents and your peers say, "Yes, do more of that. We'll sing songs about you doing that. That is what we celebrate." But if you feel same-sex attraction, your Viking culture will tell you to repress it, saying, "That is not who we are, it is not authentic, and it should not be nurtured."

People living today are told exactly the opposite: "You must suppress your impulse toward violence and nurture your same-sex attraction." Keller asks, Which culture is right? A thousand years from now, the culture

---

12. For more on the different types of love and the need for deep friendship, see C. S. Lewis's book *The Four Loves* (Mariner Books, 1971).

13. Timothy Keller, *Preaching: Communicating Faith in an Age of Skepticism* (Viking, 2015), 135–136.

will say something else. The question is, Is there something outside of culture, something that *transcends* culture, something that defines a sexual ethic, that is global, historical, and permanent? The answer, of course, is yes! God has a good plan for your sexuality if you will receive it instead of suppressing what He reveals.

Attraction

The fourth contributing factor of embracing LGBTQ+ identities is attraction. Some people experience same-sex attraction, even if they have never sought to cultivate it. It's just there, and it's always been there. Rebecca McLaughlin is a brilliant Christian author and speaker with a PhD in renaissance literature from Cambridge. She is also a wife and mother who has experienced bisexual attraction her entire life.

In her book *Confronting Christianity*, McLaughlin shares studies from Lisa Diamond (a lesbian activist), noting that while 1 percent of women are exclusively same-sex oriented, up to 14 percent have experienced attraction to both men and women at some point in their lives. Meanwhile, less than 2 percent of men are exclusively same-sex attracted, but around 7 percent have experienced attraction to both men and women.[14]

McLaughlin shares her story with both the kindness of a fellow struggler and the clarity of a faithful believer who affirms what Scripture teaches about our hearts and affections. She also agrees with one of the main premises we discussed earlier in this book: Sexual ethics are

---

14. Rebecca McLaughlin, *Confronting Christianity: 12 Hard Questions for the World's Largest Religion* (Crossway, 2019), 168.

never primarily about attraction. They are always, first and foremost, about authority.

The question is not Who or what attracts you? but rather Whose authority are you under? It doesn't matter who you are; each of us must draw a line somewhere. Even the most radical progressive will say at some point, "You shouldn't do *that*." We each must answer the question of who gets to determine which sexual attractions should be encouraged and which should be discouraged. My position, based on the truth of God's Word and the testimony of His people for two millennia, is that the God who made us and gave us gender, sexuality, and sexual activity is the sole judge of what we are to do with these good gifts.

As we consider these four factors influencing same-sex attraction and identity (abuse, addiction, attention, and attraction), it is important to keep in mind that homosexuality is not a uniform experience. Some of these factors may not be present at all, or they may exist in different proportions, person-to-person. If we're going to care about the people around us who identify this way, it's helpful to understand how they got there, because we want to be compassionate and kind.

Convictions, Not Concessions

No matter how compassionate we are, we must also be extremely clear about what we believe and what the Bible says on this issue. Homosexuality is undeniably a sin according to Scripture. Any attempt to define it otherwise is simply dishonest.

You may hear a different argument from certain "Christian" authors or pastors or podcasters. They may sound incredibly smart and sensitive. They may present what feels like a more loving approach. Their arguments may seem compelling—at first. But here's the problem: *They are not being honest.* Their argumentation assumes the conclusion they want to make. They let their desired conclusion shape how they interpret Scripture instead of letting Scripture determine their beliefs.

In his second letter to Timothy, Paul warns the young pastor to keep preaching Scripture, because

> the time will come when [people] will not endure sound doctrine, but according to their own desires, because they have itching ears, they will heap up for themselves teachers; and they will turn their ears away from the truth, and be turned aside to fables. But you be watchful in all things, endure afflictions, do the work of an evangelist, fulfill your ministry. (2 Timothy 4:3–5)

People will find someone to say what they want to hear. You may have churches like this in your community. They present themselves as welcoming and affirming, but I can almost certainly guarantee they are not known for their solid understanding and proclamation of Scripture or their high view of the Bible, because no one makes an honest attempt to read the Bible's clear passages on homosexuality, looking to the original context and intent of the authors, and concludes that Scripture permits or encourages homosexuality. No one who seeks to follow Jesus with all their heart, soul, mind, and strength is led into homosexual identity through their spiritual devotion. As James writes, "God cannot be tempted by evil, nor does He Himself tempt anyone" (James 1:13).

Instead, people experience an internal, same-sex impulse or desire and then attempt to reconcile that with following Jesus. This is true of all people who struggle with sexual sin and temptation but do not want to submit it to Jesus's authority. In a sense, they look for a way to serve two masters, and Jesus already told us that such attempts are futile (Matthew 6:24).

So how did we get to the place where people (and even some pastors and churches) are affirming of homosexuality when God's view is so clear in Scripture? The answer is that *our convictions tend to collapse in the face of close relationships and awkward conversations.*

It's challenging to hold a conviction against something when you know and love someone who embraces it. The sad truth is that many Christians are just one gay child or grandchild away from completely changing their theology on this subject. The Word of God does not change. But if our circumstances or relationships do, we are tempted to find a way to justify the change because we don't want to feel like we are condemning our friend or loved one's identity.[15]

While that is a good (or at least well-intentioned) instinct, it's still a bad conclusion. It's a good instinct to love people, even our unsaved neighbors and loved ones. They may be nice, fun, and funny. They may seek to be good people and live ethical lives, helping others and showing kindness. When you are pressed on the question of whether God really condemns your kind and welcoming

---

15. For a clear, pastoral examination of the Bible verses that directly address homosexuality and the questions people have about them, check out Kevin DeYoung's small but effective book *What Does the Bible Really Teach About Homosexuality?* (Crossway, 2015).

gay neighbor or coworker, you are tempted to hesitate. You want to support them. You don't want to be unkind or give them a bad impression of Christians. But if you are unable to say that they are wrong about their understanding of God and His authority over their lives, you are essentially saying that God's Word must be wrong about them.

Let me draw your attention back to Romans 1, pointing out something really, really hard at the end of the chapter. As we have seen already, Paul highlights sexual sin as the epitome of being given over to selfish desires, but it's not the only way we go wrong. There are many other ways:

> And even as they did not like to retain God in their knowledge, God gave them over to a debased mind, to do those things which are not fitting; being filled with all unrighteousness, sexual immorality, wickedness, covetousness, maliciousness; full of envy, murder, strife, deceit, evil-mindedness; they are whisperers, backbiters, haters of God, violent, proud, boasters, inventors of evil things, disobedient to parents, undiscerning, untrustworthy, unloving, unforgiving, unmerciful; who, knowing the righteous judgment of God, that those who practice such things are deserving of death, not only do the same but also approve of those who practice them. (Romans 1:28–32)

That last verse should make you extremely uncomfortable if you're trying to find a way to affirm someone else's sexual sin.

If you find your loyalty to this person pulling you away from your loyalty to God, I want you to know *I'm sympathetic to your dilemma.* It's a real challenge. But as a minister of the gospel, I must warn you that you *cannot* lend your approval to a sinner and still be pleasing to God. My friend, I sincerely understand if you are struggling with this idea. It may seem too difficult or unkind or harsh to accept. But remember, Jesus says really hard things too:

> Do not think that I came to bring peace on earth. I did not come to bring peace but a sword. For I have come to "set a man against his father, a daughter against her mother, and a daughter-in-law against her mother-in-law"; and "a man's enemies will be those of his own household." He who loves father or mother more than Me is not worthy of Me. And he who loves son or daughter more than Me is not worthy of Me. And he who does not take his cross and follow after Me is not worthy of Me. He who finds his life will lose it, and he who loses his life for My sake will find it. (Matthew 10:34–39)

When it comes to approving unnatural sexual identities like homosexuality and transgenderism, I understand that you want to show love to people, and I want to be sympathetic to that impulse. We should not seek to hate or harm people who are made in God's image, but that does not mean we should affirm every desire they experience or identity they wish to embrace. If we act on our momentary impulse and affirm a person's sin, it may lead to long-term harm if that person determines to remain in their sinful condition.

Rosaria Butterfield was a professor at Syracuse University and a practicing lesbian when she first heard the gospel and experienced the love of Christians who welcomed her while still clearly communicating God's design and commands regarding sexuality. Their faithful witness made a way for the Holy Spirit to transform Butterfield's life. Today, she is a mother and pastor's wife. She says the fundamental issue is not really a person's sexuality but their *pride*. No one wants to be told they're wrong and that they need to repent.[16]

Pastor and author J. D. Greear captures this point well:

> The call to repentance isn't just offensive to gay people. It's offensive to us all. Perhaps the pressing question for this generation of Christians isn't "Will we be faithful to the biblical teachings on homosexuality?" There's a more fundamental question: "Are we actually preaching repentance?" Once you've accepted you must "deny yourself" and "take up a cross" to follow Jesus, the specific things you have to give up become less significant.[17]

---

16. Rosaria Champagne Butterfield, *The Secret Thoughts of an Unlikely Convert: An English Professor's Journey into Christian Faith* (Crown & Covenant Publications, 2014), 67. You can also find more of Butterfield's writing on holy sexuality and cultural confusion in her recent book *Five Lies of Our Anti-Christian Age* (Crossway, 2023).

17. J. D. Greear, "Downplaying the Sin of Homosexuality Won't Win the Next Generation," The Gospel Coalition, February 9, 2023, https://www.thegospelcoalition.org/article/downplay-homosexual-sin-generation/.

Christian, we must call *all* people to repent who are entangled in sexual sin. And we must provide the example for what that looks like by repenting ourselves. It's the most loving thing we can do.

Born This Way, or Born Again?

OK, so here's the big question: Can someone experience same-sex attraction and still be saved? *Yes.* As a heterosexual man, I experience opposite-sex attraction to women who are not my wife from time to time, and God still lets me pastor a church. The point is, attraction alone is not sinful. But I can't take action on the attraction, and neither can the person experiencing same-sex attraction. I must submit the desires of my flesh to God, and so must they. I must live under authority, not attraction, and so must they. For most people, regardless of their sexual orientation, this will be a lifelong battle. Ask the older people you know if lust or physical desire is still an issue for them, and many will say yes, well into their advanced years. But the spiritually mature have learned to recognize it quickly and fight it effectively.

After more than sixteen years of ministry in the Washington, DC, area, I have known and talked to several people in the church who have experienced same-sex attraction. I've told them, "You're welcome here. You can serve in ministry here. I'm not as concerned about who you're *attracted* to as I am about whose *authority* you're under."

Homosexuality is not an unforgivable sin. But this is where we come back to an important principle I have highlighted throughout this book: There is a difference between temptation and sin. You may experience an attraction that you did not ask for or seek out, but it is there. It's a source of temptation to you. However, if you don't act on it or define yourself by it—if you don't feed it and nurture it—*then you have not sinned.*

If you struggle with any homosexual temptation or gender confusion, do not give up hope. Continue to seek God. He will change your heart and make you new. By His Spirit, He will help you put that desire to death. He may or may not lead you into a heterosexual relationship, but even if He does not, you can still live a life of faithful obedience with your sexuality submitted to Jesus, just like the rest of us. Pursuing holy sexuality may be hard for you, just as it is hard in similar and different ways for others. Even if you remain celibate for the rest of your life, you can still live a complete and God-glorifying life in obedience to Christ.

We have many examples of faithful people called to singleness in the Bible. John the Baptist and Daniel the prophet were unmarried, and even Jesus Himself was unmarried throughout His earthly ministry. These are some pretty heavy hitters. I doubt they looked back on their lives with disappointment or feeling as if they missed an opportunity because they didn't have a partner or were not married.

Contrary to whatever Abraham Maslow (the author of the famous "hierarchy of needs") may say, you do not need sex for survival or fulfillment.[18] What you need, more than anything, is to receive what God says as true

---

18. Abraham H. Maslow, *Motivation and Personality* (Harper & Row, 1954), 39.

and authoritative, instead of suppressing the truth, and then to lean on Him for strength to submit to His will when life is difficult.

We both have sexual temptations to fight as we walk this path of obedience. You shouldn't lust after that person of the same sex; I shouldn't lust after this person of the opposite sex. It's wrong for you to linger in your sinful desires, just as it is wrong for me to linger in mine. As Rebecca McLaughlin notes, "While we do not get to choose our sexual *attractions*, we do choose our sexual *actions*."[19] I would add that we also choose whether we will feed or starve those attractions. So let me encourage you once more: Cut out the things that make you stumble, and nurture the things that make you strong in the Lord!

And if you are tempted to give up on obedience and give in to the sinful desires and lusts you fight daily, remember that this was written to some of the first Christians in the early church:

> Do you not know that the unrighteous will not inherit the kingdom of God? Do not be deceived. Neither fornicators, nor idolaters, nor adulterers, nor homosexuals, nor sodomites, nor thieves, nor covetous, nor drunkards, nor revilers, nor extortioners will inherit the kingdom of God. And such *were* some of you. But you were washed, but you were sanctified, but you were justified in the name of the Lord Jesus and by the Spirit of our God. (1 Corinthians 6:9–11, emphasis mine)

---

19. McLaughlin, *Confronting Christianity*, 171.

Some of the very first Christians entered the church with homosexual histories and desires.[20] You are not the first and you will not be the last to have your life radically changed by God's amazing grace.

God has a good plan for us when it comes to sex and sexuality. The freedom He offers comes from living *under His authority* instead of living *by our attractions*. Our goal is to submit our sexuality to Jesus. The temptations outside of us and the rebel flesh within us are going to make that hard for almost all of us. But remember the promise we continue to hold on to throughout this book: "If we confess our sins, He is faithful and just to forgive us our sins and to cleanse us from all unrighteousness" (1 John 1:9).

---

20. McLaughlin, *Confronting Christianity*, 166.

Reflection Questions – Chapter 5

1. God is both intolerant of sin and loves to rescue sinners. How do you personally reconcile the idea of God's hatred of sin with His deep love for those who struggle with sin? How can understanding this dual aspect of God's character impact your view of your own struggles and the struggles of others?

2. This chapter discussed how cultural influences can shape our understanding of sexuality and identity. How have you seen cultural values influence perceptions of sexuality in your own life or in society? How can Christians navigate these cultural pressures while remaining true to biblical teachings?

3. How can you balance compassion and clarity when discussing sensitive issues like homosexuality with others? What are some practical ways to approach these conversations with both kindness and conviction, ensuring that you uphold biblical truth while showing love and respect?

4. There is a difference between experiencing attraction and acting on that attraction. How can understanding this distinction help you work through your own temptations and desires?

5. Consider how personal relationships can influence our theology and convictions. Have you experienced a situation in which your personal relationships affected your views on a particular issue or your willingness to address those issues? How did you navigate that situation, and what did you learn

about maintaining your biblical convictions amid personal connections?

6. J. D. Greear's quote suggests that the call to repentance is central to the Christian life. How do you understand the concept of repentance in the context of sexual sin? What does true repentance look like, and how can you encourage yourself and others to embrace it in light of these truths?

6

Escaping the Trap of Sexual Sin

I hope the main thing you take away from this book is the knowledge that you *can* change. By God's grace and with His strength, you can be set free from the bondage of sexual sin. The script for the rest of your life can be rewritten. You are not stuck.

No matter who you are or what you struggle with, change is possible with Jesus. He has been rescuing, redeeming, comforting, and strengthening people like you for thousands of years. Your sin is not the one problem He can't solve.

In this chapter, we will consider three biblical principles for breaking free from patterns and habits of sin, including sexual sin. It is important to keep in mind that these principles can be applied to other areas of life as well. The Word of God is the key to facing all of life's challenges because it contains "all things that pertain to life and godliness" (2 Peter 1:3).

When we submit to what God says in His Word about His expectations for our sexuality, we will be able to begin removing the things that poison our expectations and ideas.

The Road to Nowhere

If you've ever been in a large hotel or an airport, you have likely seen a sign posted with a map of the building, labeled with important information like the location of exits, coffee shops, and bathrooms. However, if you need to make a connecting flight, the building layout is not enough information. You also need to see a large dot that says "You are here." Recognizing your starting point helps you reach your destination.

If you are ready to change the direction of your spiritual life, you need both a trustworthy map (God's Word) and an honest understanding about where you are currently. When it comes to sexual sin, there is a path that leads to destruction, and if you want to change course, you must first recognize how far you have traveled down this path. You may find yourself in one of three stages:

- Stage 1: The wide road of sexual destruction starts with being *curious*. You are tempted by something new, something intriguing, something forbidden. You may be ambushed by it, or you may intentionally wander onto its path, but one way or another, your head is turned, your pace slows, and you linger as you look on (see Proverbs 7:6–23).

- Stage 2: Next, you begin to feel *compelled* by it. This new behavior is pleasurable and distracting. You come back to it again and again, and you begin to look forward to it. It starts to intrude on your thoughts, and you become less able to resist its siren song.

- Stage 3: Finally, you realize you are *caged* by it. You try to push away the desire, but you can't shake it. On some level, you realize you shouldn't watch that video or pursue that sexual encounter. You know it is wrong, and you fear your new habit or addiction will be discovered by others. Nevertheless, you keep going back to it. Worse, you discover that you need to push into darker and more transgressive places to experience the high you felt at first. The thought of pursuing this activity is now crowding out your other thoughts during the day, disrupting your ability to take care of other tasks.

Remember, this is a slippery slope. Sins that seem harmless and hidden still have teeth. Once they latch on to you, they won't let go easily. Your first step toward breaking free from sexual sin partly depends on where you are on this path of destruction:

- Stage 1: If you fell into something because you were bored or curious and it just got the best of you, you may simply need to repent for your misstep and get back to following Jesus.

- Stage 2: If you have begun to feel compelled by sexual temptation and sin—if you have given in to it, liked it, and begun pursuing it more and more—you will need to do some hard work to break this destructive habit and replace it with new ones.

- Stage 3: If you realize that you are caged, possibly even clinically addicted, escaping the trap is going to take some serious intervention with someone trained to help you. Being caged by a sinful addiction is the spiritual equivalent of a life-threatening illness or injury. Aside from miraculous deliverance (which you should still earnestly pray for), you're going to need more than a first aid kit; you're going to need a spiritual ICU (intensive care unit). You may need to enlist the help of a few godly friends and mentors who can get up close and personal to help you overcome the ugly outcome of this sin and begin restoring what it has damaged.

Recognizing where you are and being honest about the condition you are in is the first step toward breaking free. The second step is identifying the specific roadblocks that may be keeping you stuck.

Identifying and Navigating Roadblocks

As you travel down the path of sexual destruction, you will gather enablers along the way that accelerate and amplify the problem. When you decide to turn around and escape the trap of sexual sin, these enablers turn into roadblocks as you journey out of the darkness. I would like to discuss five of them.

Abuse

The first enabler is the issue of abuse and how its long-term effects can encourage our sin and block our escape. People don't always walk into sexual sin on their own; sometimes they are brought there by someone else. Perhaps a friend or family member showed you something or led or lured you into something without your consent and it became a part of your identity.

I know a pastor whose dad would buy him pornography magazines when he was a boy and told him he could "figure it out." I spoke with another man whose first exposure to pornography came when he was only five years old. A woman I met recently encouraged me to speak boldly about this subject because her first sexual encounter happened when she was molested at the age of seven. She's now middle-aged, but her views on the subject are still shaped by that experience.

Friend, if abuse is partly to blame for why you are where you are, know this: The gospel promises healing and recovery from the wrongs you have done *as well as the wrongs done to you*. Where you are doesn't have to define *who* you are. God created you and made you in His image, and Jesus wants to redeem and renew you. I hope you will let Him. There can be a clear turning point from who you once were to who you truly are in Christ. As Paul tells us in 2 Corinthians 5:17, "Therefore, if *anyone* is in Christ, he is a new creation; old things have passed away; behold, all things have become new" (emphasis mine). Paul's mention of "anyone" in this passage includes you, friend. As difficult as it may seem, and while healing takes time, you *can* leave behind your old self and put on your new identity in Christ Jesus.

As my old pastor used to say, "God can restore your ability to blush." He can restore your innocence. He can restore your purity so that you don't have to be defiled forever. You don't have to be defined by what you have seen or by what you have done or by what has been done to you. While you didn't choose your abuse, you can choose to let God break your chains so its effects no longer have a hold on you and can no longer propel you further into sin.

Access

The second enabler that may block our escape is access. The earliest computers were large enough to fill an entire room. Later, they were small enough to fit on a large desk or table. When I was in high school, the typical family had only one shared computer, if they had one at all. Now, computers fit in our pockets and, even though we rarely place a call with them, we call them "phones."[1] Not only that, but we live in the internet age, where literally anything we can imagine is a few clicks away. With such personal, portable access to the internet, our hearts are easily tempted to pursue their own wicked desires.

Anonymity

The snare of anonymity is the third enabler. Pornography used to be limited to magazines and films that required traveling to a certain type of store and looking a clerk in the eye in order to purchase them. Now, the supercomputer in your pocket can deliver more sexual content than an entire adult bookstore and can offer it to you in the privacy of your own home. This means you may be able to hide your sinful addiction and your search history from the people around you, at least for a while. But don't be fooled by the illusion of anonymity; no privacy blocker ever conceals you from the eyes of God. As Jesus said, "For there is nothing covered that will not be revealed, nor hidden that will not be known. Therefore

---

1. For more on this idea, check out Samuel D. James, *Digital Liturgies: Rediscovering Christian Wisdom in an Online Age* (Crossway, 2023), especially chap. 7, "Naked in the Dark."

whatever you have spoken in the dark will be heard in the light, and what you have spoken in the ear in inner rooms will be proclaimed on the housetops" (Luke 12:2–3). God knows what we do in secret, and our sin will eventually be exposed.

Approval

The fourth enabler is approval. For generations, the consumption of sexual content and use of pornography was considered sinful and undignified. Such things were never discussed in polite society, and there was a level of social stigma against illicit sexual behavior. In recent generations, though, such social barriers have begun to fall. Content that once was not allowed on the radio or on television is now commonly accepted and expected. Topics like pornography have been transformed from shameful secrets to sitcom punch lines. With the advent of video streaming services, you can find all kinds of unspeakable things on Netflix, Amazon, and YouTube. While there are still a few sexual matters considered taboo (at least in the mainstream), those boundary lines are blurring rapidly. Now, some "health professionals" actively encourage using pornography as a healthy part of one's sexuality. The month of June is set aside in popular culture and corporate America as a time to honor those who have rejected God's design for holy sexuality and who have "exchanged the natural use for what is against nature . . . committing what is shameful" (Romans 1:26–27). The moral madness of transgenderism is now mainstream, celebrated on magazine covers and at red-carpet events. There is very little in terms of sexual depravity that our modern society does not endorse.

Ambush

The fifth enabler that can be a roadblock to our escape is ambush. In other words, you don't have to go looking for opportunities to fall into sexual temptation; opportunities find you, usually when you are bored, tired, hungry, or hurt. In moments of physical and emotional weakness, we let our guard down, giving the Enemy a chance to set a trap for us. 1 Peter 5:8 tells us, "Be sober, be vigilant; because your adversary the devil walks about like a roaring lion, seeking whom he may devour."

The digital world is an attention-based economy designed to engage and enrapture you. Web designers, engineers, and app developers all want to keep you on their platforms using their programs for as long as possible. The algorithms that are designed to maximize your time of engagement online are all too eager to provide new content for you to consume, keeping you engaged and always coming back. This is how the internet is designed to work. That's why the digital marketplace is soaked in sexuality: *Sex sells*. It keeps consumers engaged the longest. The longer you wander around online without guarding your eyes and heart against temptation, the more likely you are to see things that make you curious and that entice your flesh to go down the road of destruction. The question is, Will you resist it, or will you give in? Will you click off, or will you click on? Will you let Jesus renew you and remove these roadblocks from your path? Will you let Him fight *for you* and *with you*?

That said, the third step toward breaking free from sexual sin is to recognize it as spiritual warfare needing to be fought from all angles.

A War on Multiple Fronts

In June of 1940, after Britain narrowly avoided disaster with the evacuation of Dunkirk, Prime Minister Winston Churchill delivered a stirring speech to rally Parliament and the British people. He declared that even if other nations were to fall under Nazi rule, Britain would never surrender:

> We shall go on to the end, we shall fight in France, we shall fight on the seas and oceans, we shall fight with growing confidence and growing strength in the air, we shall defend our Island, whatever the cost may be, we shall fight on the beaches, we shall fight on the landing grounds, we shall fight in the fields and in the streets, we shall fight in the hills; we shall never surrender.[2]

The determination to face a relentless evil, no matter where the battle raged, kept the British people resolute for years before the tide of the war finally turned. The nation knew they had no other option.

Since that time, the nature of warfare has changed. For thousands of years, armies fought on land, each side lining up against the other across the field of battle. Then, massive navies took imperial battles to the seas—and the best of those had Marines!

Little more than a century ago, we began to fight wars in the air as well as on the ground and in the water.

---

2. Winston Churchill, "We Shall Fight on the Beaches," speech delivered to the House of Commons, International Churchill Society, accessed February 11, 2025, https://winstonchurchill.org/resources/speeches/1940-the-finest-hour/we-shall-fight-on-the-beaches/.

Now, both physical space and cyberspace are available theaters of war in what is called "multi-domain operations." The warfare of the future is expected to be both complex and sophisticated. Free nations must bring tools, tactics, and technology to bear on a variety of fronts. We use space-based satellites for communication and observation. We use cyber warfare to attack enemy communications and defend our own. We use small, special operations forces as well as large conventional forces to fight the enemy, all while applying diplomatic, informational, and economic pressure to achieve our goals.

Spiritual warfare is no less sophisticated in the battle against temptation. When it comes to your fight against sexual temptation and your escape from the snare of sexual addiction, you must have the same kind of tenacity. As you seek to submit your sexuality to Jesus, you should be prepared to *fight this war on multiple fronts simultaneously*. Your strategy will require what I call the three A's of change: admittance, action, and allies.

Admittance

The first part of your strategy for fighting this war is to admit that any sexual activity outside of God's clear guidelines is sin. Remember the whole flow of Romans 1: God reveals truth, but people suppress it. Don't deny what you've done or what you feel. Don't try to redefine it. Often, when it comes to our sin, we take one of four approaches:

- We *minimize* it, claiming it's not that big of a deal or not that bad.

- We *maximize* it, arguing that we can't change or help ourselves. We believe the sinful habit is too hard to conquer because we have been trapped in it for too long.

- We *popularize* it, suggesting that it is not a big deal, because everyone does it.

- We *legitimize* it, justifying our actions as being acceptable under our specific circumstances.

Instead, we need to *recognize* it as a violation of God's law and as a sin against Him. We must confess our sin, turn from it, and submit ourselves to Jesus.

In order to do this, you must admit—to yourself and to Jesus—what you've done. In his book *The Death of Porn*, Pastor Ray Ortlund encourages people to do this with brutal honesty, confessing in terms that are uncomfortable but absolutely true. If you consume pornography, try describing it this way:

- Today I entertained myself with sexual exploitation.

- Today I joined in the abuse of a woman.

- Today I watched her degradation for my pleasure.

- Today I took my stand with Satan against God.[3]

Truths like these are tough, aren't they? But I suspect that, as you read these statements, you may have minimized the truth in your mind, thinking, *Oh, no, that's not*

---

3. Ray Ortlund, *The Death of Porn: Men of Integrity Building a World of Nobility* (Crossway, 2021), 26.

me. That's not what I do. If that's the case, then try to name and define what you do or have done. How would you describe it?

The goal here isn't to make you hate yourself but to help you hate your sin by seeing its true nature. You need to strip away its shiny surface and realize what's really happening underneath. Once you see that what you have done is sin that defies God's authority over your life, then you can admit it to God and repent of it.

One of the best tools you can use to aid your confession is the Psalms. Read Psalm 51, in which David confesses his sin with Bathsheba. Listen to his words and notice both his brutal honesty about his sin and his hope for mercy from God:

> Have mercy upon me, O God, according to Your lovingkindness; according to the multitude of Your tender mercies, blot out my transgressions. Wash me thoroughly from my iniquity, and cleanse me from my sin. For I acknowledge my transgressions, and my sin is always before me. (Psalm 51:1–3)

Remember also the promise we have already read from John's Epistle:

> If we confess our sins, He is faithful and just to forgive us our sins and to cleanse us from all unrighteousness. (1 John 1:9)

Whoever you are, whatever your struggle, you need to know that the same Jesus who described lust as adultery committed in the heart and who said that we should "cut off" anything in our lives that causes us to sin (Matthew 5:28–30) also died to save us from those sins. He wants to set you free and scrub you spotless today.

Jesus showed kindness to many people caught up in sexual sin. He offered them grace and forgiveness while still commanding them to repent and "sin no more" (John 8:11). He never supported them remaining in their sin, but He always looked on them with compassion. Sexual sin is not unforgivable, so admit it to yourself, admit it to God, and, finally, admit it to others.

You may remember Jason Portnoy, the Silicon Valley executive whose story I told in chapter 4. Although he is not a follower of Jesus, he was able to recognize, by God's common grace, the destruction that porn caused in his life. Part of his journey included recognizing the importance of confessing his sin to others:

> My healing—again, it's hard to generalize—my healing started when I finally started to reveal my secrets. And . . . the sooner, the better.[1]

Here's why this is important from a Christian perspective: You may have sinned against other people and need to confess that sin to them. You also may need to invite others in to help you fight for healing, resist temptation, and change direction. (If you're reading this in order to help someone else in the fight, you'll want to

---

4. Tim Ferriss, host, *The Tim Ferriss Show*, podcast, episode 600, "Jason Portnoy of PayPal, Palantir, and More—Porn Addiction, the Corrosiveness of Secrets, Healing Wounds, Escaping Shame Cycles, and Books to Change Your Life," June 15, 2022, https://tim.blog/2022/06/15/jason-portnoy/.

read my recommendations on hearing others' confessions, included at the end of this chapter.)

Action

The second strategy we must employ for fighting the war against sexual sin is to take action against it.

Central to the message of Jesus and the apostles was the call to repent of sin once having admitted to it. Repentance is not just feeling bad about what you've done; it means actively and aggressively seeking to change course. So what are you going to do differently?

It starts with developing the right mindset. Consider how Paul describes a mindset of action against sin:

- "All things are lawful for me, . . . but I will not be brought under the power of any" (1 Corinthians 6:12).

- "I discipline my body and bring it into subjection" (1 Corinthians 9:27).

- "But the fruit of the Spirit is . . . self-control" (Galatians 5:22–23).

- "Let everyone who names the name of Christ depart from iniquity" (2 Timothy 2:19).

Taking action may mean making difficult choices in the short term to avoid disaster in the long term. If you are in a dating relationship and you or your dating partner are routinely struggling with pornography use, you should seriously consider ending the relationship until the porn habit is gone. Sexual sin is a dragon that will destroy or deform your dating relationship. Kill it immediately and wait to date until you have found freedom from it. Being in a relationship will not make the problem go away; it only puts you and the other person at greater risk of falling into sexual sin. And if you are married, repeated use of pornography is adultery of the heart and a violation of your marriage covenant. Such habitual betrayal of your spouse may arguably be considered biblical grounds for divorce at some point. If that sounds like a drastic response, ask yourself if you are taking your sexual sin as seriously as you should.

So what does taking action look like practically? Let's say you are addicted to internet pornography and have admitted to God, to yourself, and to others that you need to repent and change. What now?

If you're losing the fight through temptation, you need to address the issue of access. Where, when, and how are you getting the sexually explicit material? How can you block it so that you cannot get to it and so it cannot get to you? What do you need to download, delete, or erase so the algorithms don't suggest more sexually enticing images or videos? It may take time and energy, but Jesus used imagery like cutting off your hand and plucking out your eye to describe the fight against sin (Matthew 5:28–30). He wants us to be *serious* about getting rid of it.

Paul says in Romans 13:14 that we should "make no provision for the flesh, to fulfill its lusts." This means cutting off the enemy supply lines. You might need to get a "dumb" phone that cannot access the internet. You may have to cancel a streaming service subscription, even if it provides access to other acceptable things you enjoy. It's not worth being able to discuss the latest episode of a hit show with your coworkers if you know that watching that show gives you access to sexual images and ideas that feed your lust. Cut it off—*all of it*.

Not only should you be removing sexual content from your life, but you should also be replacing it with what is holy. You want to grow both in your knowledge of Jesus and in your enjoyment of Him. You want to give your mind new things to think about and give your heart something new to desire (Philippians 4:8). Listen to how the psalmist approaches purity:

> How can a young man cleanse his way? By taking heed according to Your word. With my whole heart I have sought You; oh, let me not wander from Your commandments! Your word I have hidden in my heart, that I might not sin against You. (Psalm 119:9–11)

Holy living depends not only on avoiding sin but also on pursuing God and walking according to His commands. Instead of spending time watching porn, spend time meditating on the Word. Listen to sermons. Build a playlist of worship songs that will lift your eyes to God and fill your heart when you're feeling empty, bored, or hungry for the things you used to enjoy.

In Ephesians chapter 4, Paul uses the language of "putting off" the deeds of the flesh and "putting on" the deeds of the Spirit. Getting rid of the things that cause you to stumble is only part of the work. Once you do this, you then need to fill that space with something good, beautiful, true, and holy. I love the memorable language used by the old Puritan pastor Thomas Chalmers. He famously delivered a sermon called "The Expulsive

Power of a New Affection," saying that the best way to remove our love for worldly pleasures is to replace them with a greater, more beautiful, more powerful love for God and appreciation of His good gifts. And isn't that what you need? *Expulsive power!*[5]

Allies

The third strategy for fighting the war against sexual sin is to seek allies who will fight alongside you.

Ideally, an ally is a person of the same sex who is more spiritually mature than you are or who has fought this fight and found victory over it in Christ Jesus. You need someone who can help affirm that your old actions are sinful and then help you stay strong in resisting the temptation to slide back into your sin. He or she should be able to counsel you, challenge you, and pray for and with you. While it may be encouraging to talk to friends who are working through the same struggle, they may not be able to provide the help you need to fight well. Having an ally who is not currently struggling in this area can help you maintain perspective and lift you up when you start to slip.

This is when being connected to your local church becomes so important in your fight against sexual sin. Your brothers or sisters in your local church family can meet with you, pray with you, check in on you, and give

---

5. Thomas Chalmers, "The Expulsive Power of a New Affection," C. S. Lewis Institute, accessed March 30, 2025, https://www.cslewisinstitute.org/resources/the-expulsive-power-of-a-new-affection/.

you opportunities to confess regularly when you need to come clean. Your pastors and elders can provide counsel and support as well.

If you're married, you need to bring your spouse onto your team. These conversations may be difficult at first, but having a spouse who prays for you, supports you, and helps you take action in the fight against sin is a gift from God. You also need other allies to help keep you accountable so that your spouse does not have to bear the weight alone, so be sure to find a friend, counselor, or pastor who can help you become the man or woman your spouse needs you to be.

Above all, remember that if you confess your sin, you already have the best ally you can get. When you read the Gospels, it becomes clear that Jesus prefers the messy cases. He came to rescue you. He prays for you (Luke 22:31–32; John 17; Romans 8:26–27), promises to give you grace in your time of need (Hebrews 4:14–16), and fights for you (Exodus 14:14). You have the Holy Spirit upon you and within you. You are not alone.

You *can* escape the snare of sexual sin. Jesus came to proclaim freedom for the captives—and that includes those who are held captive by their own lusts. Call out to Him for rescue, and He will give you the strength to stand firm in your battle and break free from the chains that bind you. Admit your sin before God and your need of Him. Take action to change direction and walk in holiness. Reach out to allies who can fight alongside you. Jesus has already won your victory; it's time to take hold of it and put on your new identity in Christ. For "old things have passed away; behold, all things have become new" (2 Corinthians 5:17)!

Advice on Hearing Confessions

For those who are helping someone they love confess their sin, I offer the following advice:

- First, one of my seminary professors used to say, "You don't need to take the lid off the sewer to know that it stinks." In other words, it may be better to speak with your friend in general terms about the sexual sin they're struggling with—not so generally that the person confessing can minimize their sin but also not so specifically that you entertain impure thoughts as the hearer. Frankly, you don't need what's in their head to be in your head, and specific details usually won't change how you counsel or pray for them.

- Second, if you are the parent or spouse of the person confessing sexual sin, remember that their sin is not your fault. You can do everything possible to help guard against sin in your loved one's life, but ultimately, we are each accountable for our own actions and the desires of our hearts. Parents and spouses can help create guardrails that make it more difficult to drift into sin, but people can still lose control at any time.

- Third, I want to remind you that God sees your own sin and failures and loves you anyway, because of Jesus. Can you see this sinner's failure and love them the same way, no matter how disappointed, hurt, or shocked you are? You might need some time to process this. But remember that the same list of sins in Romans 1 that describes sexual corruption also lists being unmerciful (v. 31). When your friend or loved one confesses their sin to you, listen to them, love them, pray for and with them, and then take it all to Jesus, asking for His help.

- Fourth, remember that forgiveness is a decision, but reconciliation is a process. If you have been betrayed by your loved one's sexual sin, you may need time to process their admission. They have already thought about and processed it, so it is OK if you need time to get up to speed. Trust that is broken may be mended eventually, but it takes patience and time.

- Fifth, perhaps you already know about your loved one's sexual sin, but they are unwilling to confess it. Before confronting them, consider your goal: How do you want this to end? Do you want them to have worldly sorrow that brings only condemnation or godly sorrow that leads to repentance and change? What's the long-term goal? Will you stand with them in their fight for purity or cut them loose to fight alone? Let your desired outcome shape your initial approach.

Reflection Questions – Chapter 6

1. Reflect on the idea that "change is possible" with Jesus. What specific areas of your life do you feel need transformation? How does the promise of change through Christ encourage or challenge you?

2. We considered the path to destruction that includes the stages of curiosity, desire, and eventual addiction. Can you identify the stage of this path that you or someone you know might be in? How can recognizing these stages help bring about change?

3. What practical steps can you take to address the enablers of sin (access, anonymity, approval, ambush, or the effects of abuse)? Think of some strategies that have worked for you or that could help in the fight against temptation.

4. This chapter emphasized the importance of admitting sin to ourselves, to God, and to others. How does confessing sin openly and honestly to a trusted person or group impact the process of repentance and healing?

5. Discuss the three A's of change: admittance, action, and allies. How can you apply each of these strategies in your own life? What specific actions can you take to overcome a current struggle or temptation?

6. Who are the allies in your life who can support you in your journey of change? How can you cultivate these relationships to ensure you have a strong support system?

7. How do passages like Psalm 51 and 1 John 1:9 provide hope and guidance when addressing sin and seeking forgiveness? How can you incorporate these Scriptures into your daily life to reinforce your commitment to change?

8. Beyond immediate actions, what are some long-term practices that can help you stay aligned with God's plan for your sexuality and life overall? How can you continually seek to grow in your relationship with Jesus and remain vigilant against sin?

7
The Source of Our Sexual Struggles

In Romans 1, sexual sin is presented as the fundamental essence of choosing to walk in the flesh. I want you to stop and consider that, especially if there is any temptation toward sexual sin in your life. Of all the sins that could have been named here, sexual sin was put forward as the primary, life-marking evidence of people who have consistently and persistently suppressed the truth of God and who have been given over to wrath by Him as a result. And that sin, along with all other sin, brings death.

Friend, that should frighten us.

From the very beginning, God created man and woman with the intent that they should share a lifelong, monogamous sexual relationship. The two should become one flesh, and that which God has joined together should never be separated by anyone or anything. Men and women are to have children and live together in holy, happy harmony. Second only to their relationship with God, their exclusive relationship with each other is to be the absolute bedrock foundation of their home, life, and purpose. Holy, obedient sexuality is to be an essential component of walking in the Spirit and enjoying all the blessings God baked into the system of life.

When we step away from this path—whether through sexual activity before marriage, through sexual relationships apart from a heterosexual spouse during marriage, through seeking sexual satisfaction in pornography, or through attempting to deny how God created us by seeking to "change" our sex—we step into God's wrath.

> For the wrath of God is revealed from heaven against all ungodliness and unrighteousness of men, who by their unrighteousness suppress the truth. For what can be known about God is plain to them, because God has shown it to them. For his invisible attributes, namely, his eternal power and divine nature, have been clearly perceived, ever since the creation of the world, in the things that have been made. So they are without excuse. For although they knew God, they did not honor him as God or give thanks to him, but they became futile in their thinking, and their foolish hearts were darkened. Claiming to be wise, they became fools, and exchanged the glory of the immortal God for images resembling mortal man and birds and animals and creeping things. Therefore God gave them up in the lusts of their hearts to impurity, to the dishonoring of their bodies among themselves, because they exchanged the truth about God for a lie and worshiped and served the creature rather than the Creator, who is blessed forever! Amen. For this reason God gave them up to dishonorable passions. For their women exchanged natural rela-

tions for those that are contrary to nature; and the men likewise gave up natural relations with women and were consumed with passion for one another, men committing shameless acts with men and receiving in themselves the due penalty for their error. And since they did not see fit to acknowledge God, God gave them up to a debased mind to do what ought not to be done. They were filled with all manner of unrighteousness, evil, covetousness, malice. They are full of envy, murder, strife, deceit, maliciousness. They are gossips, slanderers, haters of God, insolent, haughty, boastful, inventors of evil, disobedient to parents, foolish, faithless, heartless, ruthless. Though they know God's righteous decree that those who practice such things deserve to die, they not only do them but give approval to those who practice them. (Romans 1:18–32 ESV)

These words, written to a church in the capital city of the Roman Empire nearly two thousand years ago, sound at times like they were written yesterday. But what do they mean? What are they telling us?

Don't miss the vital point: *Many of the problems people experience in life come from resisting what we could have known, or do know, about God.* In other words, if we want to see change in our lives and the lives of others, it's not enough to modify our bad behaviors. We must reverse course and put God back at the center. Real change happens when we stop suppressing the truth and begin to see and appreciate God Himself.

As Paul explains in Romans 1:18–32, God has revealed aspects of His character in the natural world, but many people ignore this reality.[1] They vainly seek to silence the God who speaks. They refuse the testimony of natural revelation, and, although they see things clearly, they resist learning more about this God who is calling out to them.

There is a sense in which we all know only as much about God as we're willing to know. To put it another way, *we all know a little bit more about God than we wish we did*. We tend to think of "rejecting God" as hearing a clear presentation of the gospel (perhaps something like the Four Spiritual Laws[2]) and then rejecting it. But maybe it's like reading Scripture and then deciding that what it clearly says just isn't for us.

According to this passage, rejection of God's revelation is not just a rejection of Jesus as Savior; it is a rejection of God as Creator. When we reject God's revelation, we aren't simply saying, "I don't need You to save me."

---

1. Theologians speak of natural or general revelation and special or specific revelation. Special or specific revelation is received through the person of Jesus Christ and through Scripture, which was penned by prophets, apostles, and other holy men of God who "spoke as they were moved by the Holy Spirit" (2 Peter 1:21). Natural revelation occurs as God reveals truths about Himself through creation around us and conscience within us. "The heavens declare the glory of God; and the firmament shows His handiwork. . . . Their [sound] has gone out through all the earth, and their words to the end of the world" (Psalm 19:1, 4).

2. Bill Bright, *Have You Heard of the Four Spiritual Laws?* (New Life Publications, 2016). The Four Spiritual Laws are a tool for evangelism created by Bill Bright, the founder of Campus Crusade for Christ (now Cru). It presents the core message of Christianity in four key points: God's love, humanity's problem, Jesus Christ's solution, and the personal response required to experience a relationship with God. It has been widely used in personal evangelism and outreach efforts to help people understand the basics of the Christian faith.

The Source of Our Sexual Struggles

We are rejecting the very fact that God made us and has any claim on us and our lives at all.

We are made to be worshippers, but rather than worshipping the God who has revealed Himself through His creation, we suppress that truth and worship something else. We give ourselves over to the worship of created things. Our misplaced worship corrupts our thinking (Romans 1:21–23), deforms our sexuality (Romans 1:24–27), and rots our relationships with others (Romans 1:28–32).

The Great Physician, who knows our condition well, has given us His diagnosis here in Romans 1, in stark and unavoidable terms. The reason why our world is sick, full of strife, and riddled with sexual and relational brokenness is because we and all the other children of Adam have broken it. And the result of our rebellion and suppression of the truth has begun to be revealed from heaven: the righteous wrath of a holy God.

As people consistently and persistently choose to put themselves and their desires first, God eventually *gives them over to those desires*—an idea we find repeated three times in Romans 1. It's sad but true: People can resist God only for so long.

Eventually, He lets them go completely. This pattern is repeated throughout Scripture. People harden their hearts against God and His ways, and eventually, God gives them what they want. He leaves them alone to embrace the darkness. Pharaoh in the story of the Exodus is probably the most well-known example of this, but there are others.

When God does this, the outcome is not what people expect. The phrase "gave them up to" in the original Greek implies being put into the custody of another, similar to how a judge hands over a convicted criminal to the bailiff and then to the warden. When God "gives us up" to our sin, we are not set free to enjoy the "freedom" that self-rule promises; instead, we are bound by even heavier chains.

A person who has been given over to their sin cannot find lasting joy, peace, and satisfaction in it. Instead, they are driven to consume themselves and others in the never-ending search to satisfy the hunger and thirst in their souls. In Romans 1:24–27, we see that such people will devote themselves to sexual pleasure in their pursuit of satisfaction. However, rather than experiencing the joy and intimacy of holy sexuality within the bounds of godly marriage, sex itself becomes another god to worship and serve in the place of the Creator.

Not only does sexual satisfaction remain fleeting and disappointing, but God further gives them up to a corrupted mind and rotten relationships. In verses 28–32, we see the bitter fruit of that further hardening of the heart. Relationships become transactional and riddled with distrust the further and further away we move from the life and community that God intended for us. There's only one way to describe the condition of someone who has walked according to the flesh and reaped its rueful rewards: *They're under God's wrath.*

God's Wrath Revealed

When you consider the wrath of God, you may think of fire and brimstone raining from the heavens. To some, God's wrath may seem an outdated or backward idea from a more primitive version of religion. After all, doesn't the Bible say that "God is love"? Isn't He supposed to be gentle and kind? Surely, no matter how badly we mess up, if we are basically good people, He will give us a break and let us into heaven anyway, right? That's a very popular concept of how we can relate to God. Unfortunately, it's also incomplete, inaccurate, and unbiblical.

The Bible describes the character of God as embodying both perfect justice and perfect mercy. He is described in various places as a God of both wrath and grace. And if we could see the full reality of sin and its effects, we wouldn't want it any other way.

We all want justice. When someone sins against us, we want them to be punished. We want things to be made right. But what happens when *we* sin? Suddenly, we want to find a loophole in God's justice. We want our own sins to be understood, overlooked, and excused. We love justice when it benefits us but clamor for mercy when we stand guilty ourselves.

God's character does not shift the way ours does. He is and always has been perfect in His judgments and resolute in His justice, and the outcome of that justice can rightly be described as holy, just, and deserved wrath. Biblically, God's wrath can be described in three key ways: It is a righteous response to evil, a withholding of potential blessings, and a present and future reality.

A Righteous Response to Evil

When we talk about God's wrath, it is important to remember that God is not like we are. Our anger is reactive. We are quick to boil over and often easily provoked. The Bible gives us a different picture of God's wrath. He doesn't throw a temper tantrum or act in a fickle or spiteful way. When God displays His wrath and anger against evil, it is a righteous response.

God often shows patience in demonstrating His wrath. When He reveals His name to Moses in Exodus 34, He uses several traits to describe who He is. One of those traits is *longsuffering,* meaning that He is slow to anger (Exodus 34:6). Peter later writes that the apparent delay in God's final judgment isn't "slackness" or inactivity on God's part but rather a gracious patience intended to allow sinners to repent (2 Peter 3:9).

That said, we dare not seek to take advantage of the Lord's patience. Just because God is not reactive doesn't mean His burning anger isn't terrifying. In Psalm 21:9, David says of God's enemies, "The LORD shall swallow them up in His wrath, and the fire shall devour them." The writer of Hebrews later warns that "it is a fearful thing to fall into the hands of the living God" (Hebrews 10:31).

Theologian John Stott defines the wrath of God as "His holy hostility toward evil, His refusal to condone it or come to terms with it, His just judgment on it."[3] While God's nature is holy love at its center, that love is also perfectly expressed as wrath against wickedness. If there is no wickedness, there is no need for wrath. Wrath is a righteous response to the devastation and destruction brought about by sin.

A Withholding of Potential Blessings

The wrath of God is expressed not only as an active opposition to rebellion but also a withholding of the good that is available in obedience.

---

3. John R. W. Stott, *The Message of Romans,* rev. ed. (IVP Academic, 2020), 72.

All people, regardless of their decisions, experience some manner of blessing by living in the world God has created: blessings like family, food, and the simple pleasures of life. Theologians refer to these daily blessings as "common grace." Paul writes that the goodness of God to all mankind is one of the things that should lead us to repentance (Romans 2:4).

Along with common grace, we can enjoy blessings that come from walking in step with the Spirit and following the path God has designed for our lives. Often, when we align ourselves with God's commands and adhere to His design, our lives tend to function more smoothly. Think of it as the difference between swimming with the current or against it, or as a plane flying with the jet stream behind it rather than in front of it. How much extra fuel does a jet engine consume when flying against the jet stream? How much more effort must a swimmer exert to move against the sea's current?

We add unnecessary strain and difficulty to our daily lives when we are constantly at odds with God's design and commands. Instead of walking in integrity, we lie and cheat others, forcing ourselves to maintain and compound those lies to avoid discovery. We abuse and mistreat people, which breeds more anger, bitterness, distrust, and strife in our relationships. We seek validation and fulfillment in created things, but when they disappoint us, we are left with an empty void. It doesn't have to be this way, but we inevitably reap the bitter consequences of disobedience. God ensures that the path of the sinner is hard.

That's not to say that a believer's life is easy, but we can endure life's difficulties more successfully when we align our lives with God's plans. Unfortunately, even when aligned with God, Christians face troubles from other sources: from interacting with other sinners, contending with a demonic Enemy who opposes us, and living on a broken planet where challenges are inevitable. These consequences of the Fall sweep through our lives, attempting to push us off course. While God is not the immediate source of these challenges, He will still sovereignly guide them in a believer's life to test and strengthen our faith as we rely on Him.

A Present and Future Reality

In Romans 1:18, Paul writes that "the wrath of God *is revealed* from heaven against all ungodliness and unrighteousness of men" (emphasis mine). The grammar here is in the present tense. This is happening right now. As we have seen, a life under wrath looks like a life filled with the kinds of sin listed in Romans 1. It begins fundamentally with sexual sin but includes all kinds of other harmful practices, from outward violence to inward pride. These sins not only separate us from a holy and righteous God, but they also make life increasingly difficult for other people and for ourselves.

This is the wrath of God, and it's a terrible way to live. It's the path of daily splinters leading to an eternity of suffering. In the end, this path of wrath leads to a final and eternal experience of God's wrath: the permanent removal of His blessings in judgment and hell. Paul describes this as "the wrath to come" in 1 Thessalonians 1:10. Jesus describes hell as "everlasting punishment," an "everlasting fire prepared for the devil and his angels"

(Matthew 25:41, 46). Without God's gracious intervention, this is the destiny of all people. All of us have sinned and fallen short of the glory of God (Romans 3:23), and the wages of our sin is death (Romans 6:23).

We're experiencing judgment right here, right now, and it looks like sexual immorality, violence, pride, anger, and lying. Mankind is reaping the consequences of walking according to the flesh. These behaviors that come from suppressing the truth and ignoring God inevitably end friendships, break up families, erode communities, and destroy nations. They lead us to experience wrath.

For every one of us, this is really bad news. But there is good news!

If you are walking in the flesh, God makes it possible for you to reverse course. He offers a way to cleanse you from your corruption, pull out the splinters, heal your wounds, and give you a new heart. He can rescue you from the darkness you have embraced and bring you into the Kingdom of His Son. He can set you on the path of blessing, walk with you, guide you, and give you the strength you need to keep going.

All of this is made possible through the gospel, the word that literally means "the good news." This was the message that the apostle Paul was excited to share with people in Rome in Romans 1:

> For I am not ashamed of the gospel of Christ, for it is the power of God to salvation for everyone who believes, for the Jew first and also for the Greek. For in it the righteousness of God is revealed from faith to faith; as it is written, "The just shall live by faith." (Romans 1:16–17)

Although mankind rejected God's authority as Creator and suppressed the truth in their hearts, God in His mercy made a way for men and women to be restored. He continues to call out to us to repent of our sins and come to Him through faith in Jesus. If we do that, He will forgive us, deliver us from His holy wrath, and invite us into the life of blessing that comes from being with Him.

Don't miss this part, though: God doesn't do this by ignoring our sin or waving it away. The power of the gospel is that *our sin is atoned for by Jesus*.

Remember, one of God's character traits is that He is perfectly just, and His holy justice demands that all lawbreaking and rebellion must be punished. However, rather than leave us in the darkness of sin and death, Jesus Christ stepped into our sin-soaked world, lived the perfect life of holy obedience we never could, and then willingly received the punishment for sin that was owed to us. That's what the cross is all about: The wrath and justice of God was satisfied when it was poured out on Jesus instead of being poured out on us. In Romans 3, Paul describes it this way:

> But now the righteousness of God apart from the law is revealed, being witnessed by the Law and the Prophets, even the righteousness of God, through faith in Jesus Christ, to all and on all who believe. For there is no difference; for all have sinned and fall short of the glory of God, being justified freely by His grace through the redemption that is in Christ Jesus, whom God set forth *as a propitiation by His blood, through faith, to demonstrate His righteousness*, because in His

forbearance God had passed over the sins that were previously committed, to demonstrate at the present time His righteousness, *that He might be just and the justifier* of the one who has faith in Jesus. (Romans 3:21–26, emphasis mine)

Jesus's sacrifice was the "propitiation" of our sins: the sacrifice that covered sin and satisfied God's wrath. God did this so that His justice would be upheld and so that He may justify, or declare "not guilty," all who repent and believe in Jesus. It's a pretty good deal: Your wrongs are forgiven, and you're invited into the stream of blessing. The life of blessing is made possible by the substitutionary atonement of Jesus.

The question is this, friend: Where do you stand before God right now? Are you walking according to the flesh, fulfilling its desires, or are you walking in the Spirit, obeying His commands? Have you repented, turning from your sin and putting your faith in Jesus as your substitute, sacrifice, and Savior? Are you under the blessings of God or under His wrath? You can turn back and find forgiveness and restoration today.

If you have been born again, there may still be some things in your life that are deserving of God's wrath, such as sinful attitudes and behaviors that suppress the truth and worship the created thing instead of the Creator. If that is the case, it's time to come clean. Apply the same gospel that saved you to the specific issues that plague you. Ask God to forgive you. Repent, turning away from your sin, and ask God to guide you by His Word and His Spirit into the life that Jesus is calling you to. Choose the splinter-free life of blessing from walking with God. It's available to you. It's the life God always wanted you to have.

Stepping into the Light

If we want to change what is happening in our lives, there's a clear path out of the consequences. We just have to work our way backward up the chain of events in Romans 1. Instead of suppressing the truth about God, we need to *embrace it*. Romans 1:21 says that people knew the truth about God, but they "did not glorify Him as God, nor were thankful, but became futile in their thoughts, and their foolish hearts were darkened." Like Jesus said, the light came into the world, but we all loved the darkness because our deeds were evil.

If you want to reverse course, start by embracing the light and letting it drive the darkness out of your foolish heart. Instead of becoming futile in your thoughts, accept with gratitude the truth that Scripture reveals. Instead of ignoring or resisting God, glorify Him, thank Him, turn to Him, and embrace Him. Receive the truth God is revealing instead of suppressing it.

If you want to be freed from your sexual immorality (no matter what it looks like), you're not going to find full and lasting freedom by just telling yourself to quit. You find freedom by confessing your sin, admitting it is sin, and turning to God—not just to find forgiveness but also to find a new path in life. God doesn't slap your hand and say, "Stop that!" He says, "Walk this way. Come close to Me. Be in the light. Explore what I reveal. Receive the truth and don't suppress it."

God has revealed Himself—through creation, through Scripture, and, finally and fully, through His Son. Whether you admit it or not, you have heard God's voice, been nudged by His Spirit, and been pricked by your conscience. God doesn't *have* to do any of that. But He does. How will you respond?

Don't remain in darkness any longer. The apostle John says, "If we walk in the light as He is in the light, we have fellowship with one another, and the blood of Jesus Christ His Son cleanses us from all sin" (1 John 1:7). That's how you avoid the wrath of God. That's how you change your life. That's how you find forgiveness that covers your sins, fully, freely, and forever: You begin walking in the light.

Reflection Questions – Chapter 7

1. Why do you think sexual sin is highlighted in Romans 1 as a significant indicator of walking in the flesh? How can we address issues of sexual sin compassionately and biblically?

2. In what ways, or about what, are you most likely to suppress the truth? In what area is your thinking most often faulty? In what ways is your heart dark? How do you resist the truth?

3. How do you understand the concept of walking in the Spirit versus walking in the flesh? Can you share specific examples from your life where you've experienced one path over the other?

4. Discuss the idea that God's wrath is a reaction to wickedness rather than an emotional outburst. How does this perspective change our understanding of God's character and His relationship with humanity?

5. How does understanding the gospel as both a message of salvation and a means of sanctification impact your faith? In what ways can we apply the gospel to our daily struggles?

6. What are some practical ways you can "walk in the light" of Jesus? What practices have been helpful to you in the past?

If we confess our sins, He is faithful and just to forgive us our sins and to cleanse us from all unrighteousness.
—1 John 1:9

Appendix A:
Common Questions and Answers

In this section, I want to address some common questions I've received regarding the issues addressed in this book. My hope is that the following pages can give you a little more help in finding the answers you need.

A Question on Getting Specific Help

Where should I go to get specific help?

I often tell people that, as a local church pastor, I am the spiritual equivalent of a family doctor. I can help with general guidance, spiritual care, and biblical truth. However, if you need the spiritual equivalent of an ACL repair, a kidney transplant, or chemotherapy, I'm not your guy. In those cases, I need to refer you to someone more specialized. Spiritually speaking, that means pointing you to people whose training and experience focus on particular areas of need.

For example, as a pastor, I might help my church pray through and discern whether or not to begin a building project. But once the decision is made, I'll rely on the expertise of architects and contractors to carry it out. In the same way, thoughtful Christians may begin with spiritual reflection on the issues affecting their lives, assisted by their pastors, and then move forward with help from trained professionals in other fields.

What follows is a general guide regarding different people you might turn to for help with specific issues. Of course, these are broad categories. Some individuals may be able to speak meaningfully into areas beyond their primary field, such as a Christian physician with a deep understanding of ethics or a pastor with years of experience helping people with addiction. These people are a gift when you find them, but they are the exception rather than the rule. The following is a summary of what you can expect from different kinds of counsel. Note that any specific issue you work through with a pastor, for example, could also be something to work through with a counselor and vice versa.

Pastoral Counsel
Life is inherently theological. This means that theological reflection should be the foundation for all areas of life—from our relationships and careers to our finances, health, and emotional well-being. A pastor helps you understand God's position on an issue and offers guidance for aligning your life accordingly. Your pastor should help you lay the theological foundation for the issue and then allow other specialists to help you build on that foundation. You should seek pastoral support and biblical counseling for the following issues:

- a biblical understanding of marriage and sexuality
- premarital counseling

Appendix A: Common Questions and Answers

- marriage dynamics, roles, and enrichment
- marriage after divorce and/or with blended families
- managing a spouse or partner's acute, chronic, or end-of-life health conditions
- moral decision-making (e.g., the ethics and use of in vitro fertilization [IVF])
- communicating with others
- forgiveness and reconciliation
- guilt and shame related to sexuality
- behavioral addiction (e.g., pornography or gambling)
- struggles with sexual sin
- spiritual support and guidance for major life transitions
- faith-based approaches for mental health (e.g., prayer, Scripture reading and meditation, Christian community, periods of retreat, small group Bible study)
- developing a theology of grief and loss

Professional Counsel

Mental health professionals have different titles (therapist, counselor, psychologist, etc.) as well as varying backgrounds and approaches. Think of physical fitness as a parallel: A "fitness trainer" might have a strong background in Zumba, spinning, powerlifting, yoga, cross-training, or endurance events. The challenge is finding someone whose background and approach match your fitness goals. If you want to deadlift five hundred pounds, you probably don't want to go to someone who provides training for triathlons. Similarly, you should search for a credentialed therapist who understands your goals and has experience counseling people in your situation. One might seek mental health treatment/therapy regarding the following:

- suicidal/self-harm ideation or behaviors
- mental health symptoms (post-traumatic stress disorder, depression, anxiety, as well as persistent and severe mental health disorders)
- learning about sexual response cycles and developing healthy sexual ethics
- sexual disorders
- sexual trauma
- domestic abuse/violence
- substance abuse
- behavioral addiction (e.g., pornography or gambling)
- navigating family-of-origin dynamics/communication/attachment
- managing a spouse or partner's acute or chronic health conditions
- premarital counseling
- marriage after divorce and/or blended families
- conflict resolution skills
- processing grief and loss
- life transitions

Medical Counsel

Talking to an experienced medical provider is the best option for issues related to your anatomy, bodily functions, and current or future use of medications. In some cases, you may need to get a referral from your primary doctor to see a specialist, such as a gynecologist, urologist, endocrinologist, pelvic floor physical therapist, and so on. Reasons to seek medical assessment and treatment include the following:

- questions related to birth control options or fertility
- pain during sex or loss of sexual function
- frequent urinary tract infections, especially after intercourse
- screening and treatment of sexually transmitted infections
- changes in lubrication, erectile dysfunction, premature ejaculation, anorgasmia (inability to achieve orgasm), or low sex drive
- postpartum and perimenopausal/postmenopausal sexual health changes
- mental health medication
- exploring and addressing possible underlying causes of mental health/libido/energy difficulties, including
    - ◊ thyroid
    - ◊ male and female hormone levels
    - ◊ age-related changes
    - ◊ perinatal and perimenopausal/postmenopausal changes
    - ◊ chronic illness/pain

Questions About What the Bible Says

Does the biblical definition of *fornication* include premarital sex, even if it is in a loving relationship?

Behind the English word *fornication* is the Greek word *porneia*, also translated as "sexual immorality." So, yes, the biblical definition of *fornication* includes premarital sex, even in a loving relationship. For more on this, see chapter 1, "Sex Is a Gift, Not a God," as well as the next question, below.

What is the definition of the Greek word *porneia*?

Porneia has a broad range of meanings covering many forms of sexual activity considered immoral or socially unacceptable, including prostitution, adultery, fornication, incest, or homosexuality. The term is based in the root word *pornos*, or "male prostitute," and *pernēmi*, meaning "to sell." It originally had connotations of prostitution in Greek culture but expanded to denote any sexual conduct outside the bounds of accepted norms, particularly in Jewish and Christian ethical frameworks.

Why did so many people in the Old Testament have concubines and multiple wives?

Several of the most significant male figures in the Old Testament had concubines and/or multiple wives, leading us to ask, Was this acceptable? The answer is clearly no. The Bible does two things in this regard: At times, it *describes* what is happening, and at other times, it *prescribes* what should occur. Just because we read something in Scripture that took place historically does not automatically mean we should follow the example; it may have been a negative example. In the case of multiple wives, we see that God allowed the situation to occur, but He never endorsed or blessed it. In fact, He warned against it. Long before Israel ever had a king, God warned in Deuteronomy 17:17, "Neither shall he multiply wives for himself, lest his heart turn away." Later, we read of Solomon, the third king of Israel, "And he had seven hundred wives, princesses, and three hundred concubines; and his wives turned away his heart" (1 Kings 11:3). God used these men despite their sin, and today He often does the same thing. Without endorsing the sin in our lives, God uses us to accomplish His purposes.

Questions About Restoration and Change

I've seen things, done things, and experienced things sexually that have defiled my mind. Can God restore my innocence?

Yes, absolutely! It's true that innocence, purity, and virginity are precious things that should be protected. At the same time, the Bible assures us there is nothing that has been broken that God cannot fix. One of my favorite Scriptures related to this truth is tucked away in the small Old Testament book of Joel. The prophet Joel promises the people of Israel that if they turn from their sins and seek God again, a time will come when He "will restore . . . the years that the swarming locust has eaten" (Joel 2:25). You will need to train your mind in new ways to think, though. When you start remembering those things of the past, rush to God's promises for you instead. Put off the "old you," and put on the thoughts that God wants to fill you with. Explore passages like Ephesians 4:20–24, Philippians 4:8, and Colossians 3:1–17.

I'm scared of falling back into sexual sin. How can I trust God to redeem me?

Not all fear is bad. Sometimes, fear can be an alarm sounding in our soul, saying, "Danger! Pay attention!" God doesn't want you terrified, but we are warned in Scripture to be sober-minded and alert to the dangers around us. You could fall back into sexual sin. So let that fear drive you closer to God, who will shepherd you and keep you. There's a world of difference between a child walking alone in a dangerous place and walking in the same place with a father who has spent twenty years in the Special Forces. The father's presence gives the child confidence and assurance that things are going to be OK. So stay close to your Shepherd. Don't trust in yourself, but trust in Him. He will lead you into growth and maturity, even if it's hard at times. See 1 Corinthians 10:13.

People in my life are still struggling with my past sexual immorality. How can I forgive myself and move forward?

Forgiving yourself will be bound up tightly with repentance and reconciliation. It is imperative that you first confess your sins to God and find forgiveness from Him. Then, when possible, share the news of your repentance with the people in your life who are struggling with what you have done. If appropriate, ask for their forgiveness as well. Then preach the gospel to yourself regularly. Remember: "If we confess our sins, He is faithful and just to forgive us our sins and to cleanse us from all unrighteousness" (1 John 1:9). Spend lots of time soaking in Romans 8, especially verse 1 and verses 31–34.

Appendix A: Common Questions and Answers

If a man has been exposed and addicted to porn for a long time, could that contribute to physical afflictions like erectile dysfunction? If he repents and asks Jesus to lead him and cleanse him of this sin, can erectile dysfunction be reversed? If Jesus chooses not to heal this man, what would the Lord be trying to teach him other than the fact that sin kills? What should our attitude be?

There is no doubt that our sins have consequences. I have no problem believing that there are multiple mechanisms behind those consequences. So could something like erectile dysfunction be directly related to abuse of pornography? I think it's possible. Did this occur as a spiritual corrective act of discipline, or did it happen through physiological mechanisms? I don't know. Whatever the case, I would tell you that yes, God can bring healing in both domains. First and foremost, you need to address the condition of your soul. Repent of your sins and find forgiveness in Christ. This may lead to physical healing. But if not, I encourage you to seek qualified medical help and ask God to bring you healing that way.

Ultimately, the eternal security of our soul is the most important thing. Fortunately, that security can be attained instantly through repentance in Christ. Physiological healing may also come instantly, or it may take time, or previous function may never be restored. Regardless of the timing, physical healing is always of secondary importance to spiritual restoration. I believe Jesus was speaking in hyperbole when He said to cut off your hand or pluck out your eye if it causes you to sin (Matthew 5:27–30), but the exaggeration was intended to make a point: Sin really is that big of a deal and should be dealt with radically. As Jesus says, it is better for part of your body to suffer physically than for your whole body to be cast into hell, resulting in physical *and* spiritual death.

Questions About Relationships/Divorce

What does *adultery* mean in the Bible? Does it mean only having an affair? Is having an affair the only condition God allows for divorce? What about abandonment (physical or emotional)? What about violence?

Adultery in the Bible means the same thing as it does today—having sexual relations with someone who is not your spouse. It is soundly condemned throughout the Bible (see especially Matthew 5:32, 1 Corinthians 6:9–10, and Hebrews 13:4). When Jesus addresses the issue of divorce, He states that the only clear grounds for it is fornication (*porneia*; see the earlier section "Questions About What the Bible Says").

When abandonment is the issue, the remaining Christian spouse can and should turn first to God for comfort and guidance and then reach out to their local church for help and support. When considering how to respond to abandonment, keep in mind that divorce is not a requirement. In fact, divorce is never a requirement, even for fornication. The determination of whether or not to pursue divorce on any of these grounds should be made in close consultation with people who love God and love you; who have a deep, clear understanding of all the relevant details; and who are praying with you and for the situation.

Appendix A: Common Questions and Answers

If violence is involved, the abused spouse should immediately seek to separate themselves from the abuser; there is no obligation to endure abuse. Consider how often Paul escaped harmful situations as a missionary (Acts 22:25–29; Acts 23:12–24; 2 Corinthians 11:32–33). The abused spouse should also seriously consider reporting the situation to civil authorities. Once the safety of the abused spouse and any dependent children is established, only then can they think clearly about the issue of divorce.

Is pornography use a legitimate reason for divorce?

It may be. Jesus said that to look after a woman lustfully is like committing adultery with her in your heart (Matthew 5:27–28). However, there are many issues to be explored here. For example, does the sinning spouse truly see this as a sin? Are they repentant? Is this something they fall into or freely engage in? Are they willing to confess their sin to others and seek help? As the spouse who has been sinned against, are you just as concerned about the condition of your spouse's soul as you are about feeling humiliated, betrayed, and embarrassed? As mentioned previously, the question of whether or not to pursue divorce on these grounds should be made in close consultation with people who love God and love you; who have a deep, clear understanding of all the relevant details; and who are praying with you and for the situation.

Is it possible to sin sexually in marriage?

Yes. See the sections "The Purpose of Sex" and "God-Glorifying Sex: Frequency and Form" back in chapter

3, "Passionate, Pleasant, and Pure." Sexual intercourse is given to couples as a celebration of intimacy. If the desires or actions of one spouse are bent or twisted in a way that is self-seeking at the cost of the dignity, pleasure, comfort, or conviction of the other spouse, they are likely not pleasing to God. Marriage does not provide a sanctifying cover for every desire that arises in the human heart, and spouses should not feel obligated or coerced into activities that go against their prayer-soaked conscience.

Is it acceptable to live with someone of the opposite sex if you are not sexually active?

At the very least, it probably is not wise in most situations. According to Colossians 1:22, Jesus's goal is "to present you holy, and blameless, and above reproach in His sight." If people see you and an opposite-sex roommate living together, they will likely assume you are sleeping together. If the reason for the arrangement is primarily financial, it would be wiser to find a roommate of the same sex. On the other hand, if there is a romantic interest between you, then why not wait to live together until you're married? If you're putting off marriage due to financial issues, tax issues, or health care benefits, why not take a step toward righteousness in faith and trust God for His provision? An unmarried couple of the opposite sex living together is not sinful by default, but in many cases, it would simply be unwise.

Appendix A: Common Questions and Answers

Questions About Parenting

How can we help protect our sons from the dangerous snare of pornography?

Talk to them about it, talk to God about them, and take action as wise shepherds. We must talk to both our sons and our daughters about the dangers of pornography. The book of Proverbs contains wisdom from a father to his son (the phrase "My son" occurs twenty-three times in the book), including several warnings about avoiding sexual temptation. We need to talk about these things with our kids in age-appropriate terms. We need to be open and honest about our own struggles and experiences and encourage them with the truth of the gospel when they fail. We also need to talk to God about our kids and intercede for them. This battle, like all others, is primarily spiritual in nature (Ephesians 6:12). Finally, we can also take practical steps to make it more difficult for pornography to ensnare our kids by putting safeguards around their use of technology.

How can a man who has stumbled and struggled with temptation send a message to youth without looking like a hypocrite?

Your past doesn't disqualify you, especially if you own it. Can you say honestly, "I want to keep you from the things that hurt me"? The apostle Paul calls himself the "chief" of sinners in 1 Timothy 1:15, but he then goes on to say in verse 16, "However, for this reason I obtained mercy, that in me first Jesus Christ might show all longsuffering, as a pattern to those who are going to believe on Him for everlasting life." You look like a hypocrite only if there hasn't been any change or if you pretend you have no sin. If you have repented and found new life in Christ, you are a trophy of grace and have a testimony to what grace and change look like.

How do we teach our daughters about the dangers of dressing to show off?

Talk to them about it, talk to God about them, and take action as wise shepherds, just as you should in warning your children about pornography.

I have a daughter, and we talk about these things. We also talk about the fact that wearing showy clothing isn't limited to sexually provocative clothing and that it's not just girls who do it. All people need to ask themselves, *Why am I wearing this? Am I trying to draw attention to myself? If so, what need am I trying to fulfill?* We talk about the fact that physical beauty lasts only for a season and could be gone in an instant due to an accident or injury, while spiritual beauty can grow deeper and stronger all throughout life. You should also talk to God about your daughter. Pray for her, asking God to help her know her worth in His eyes. Ask Him to make her confident in her identity regardless of how she looks or who looks at her (1 Peter 3:3–4). Then, practically, consider what clothes you're buying for her. You may decide to allow certain clothes to be worn around the house for comfort, having different criteria for what is worn outside the house—adults included.

Appendix A: Common Questions and Answers

Questions About Homosexuality

Are gay people "born that way"?

Maybe, but it's hard to know for sure. Even if they are, they don't all stay that way. In her book *Confronting Christianity*, Rebecca McLaughlin shares her own experience of same-sex attraction as well as that of a friend's, highlighting their different experiences and outcomes over the course of their lives. In her chapter titled "Isn't Christianity Homophobic?," she also cites a journal article by Lisa Diamond (a psychology professor and lesbian activist) and Clifford Rosky. In their research, the authors conclude that "arguments based on the immutability of sexual orientation are unscientific, given what we now know from longitudinal, population-based studies of naturally occurring changes in the same-sex attractions of some individuals over time."[1]

As emphasized by the title of this book, *Authority over Attraction*, the question is never simply "What am I attracted to?" but rather "What do I do with that attraction?" and "Who gets to shape my sexual ethics?" For more on this subject, see chapter 5, "Against Nature," as well as McLaughlin's book, which addresses this and other critiques of Christian sexual ethics.

---

1. Rebecca McLaughlin, *Confronting Christianity: 12 Hard Questions for the World's Largest Religion* (Crossway, 2019), 169; Lisa M. Diamond and Clifford J. Rosky, "Scrutinizing Immutability: Research on Sexual Orientation and U.S. Legal Advocacy for Sexual Minorities," *The Journal of Sex Research* 53, nos. 4–5 (2016): 363–391, https://doi.org/10.1080/00224499.2016.1139665.

Isn't Romans 1 merely a prohibition against unrestrained lust and not against loving, same-sex relationships?

No. To be as clear as possible, the Bible never promotes or condones any kind of homosexual behavior. No one seeks God, submits fully to His desires, and then experiences Him leading them into a homosexual relationship. Instead, once someone decides to give in to their homosexual desires, they often find some way to say, "While the Bible might condemn certain kinds of homosexuality, it doesn't condemn *this* kind" (by which they mean "*my* kind" or "the kind embraced by a person I love"). Most people in this camp have a direct, personal relationship with someone who experiences same-sex attraction, and often it's a friend or their child. I affirm their impulse to love their friend or child, but when God demonstrated His love for us, He did not do it by excusing our sin. Rather, He did it by rebuking our sin, calling us to repentance, and making a way for our salvation. See Kevin DeYoung's book *What Does the Bible Really Teach About Homosexuality?* for a chapter-length response to this question.

Questions About Purity

How would you respond to someone who has become self-righteous about their purity?

First, I would talk to God about the issue and ask Him to bring the person conviction and, if necessary, to open the door for me to say something in a spirit of love. Then I would talk to them about their sin, just as I would talk to anyone else about any other sin. I would also warn them that just because they have maintained their purity does not mean they're guaranteed to meet and marry someone else who has had the same experience. What if God wanted them to meet and marry someone who already had a child? I know of a couple who could not have children of their own, but one of them had a child from a previous relationship. That child became their only child for many years. It is good to work to preserve your own purity, but the motivation for this should be to please God, not to accomplish a quest. When the day for marriage comes, we should want whatever God has determined is best for us, no matter the other person's background or experience.

What would you say to someone who thinks they have "done everything right" and now expects God to do something for them?

This is not an uncommon experience. There is often a temptation to view our relationship with God as transactional. We may act as if we can lock Him into a contract: "If I do this, then God needs to do that." This misses the whole point of the gospel and of grace. It also exposes our idolatry because it shows that we don't really worship God—we worship the thing we're trying to get via God. I would talk to this person about what it means to suffer for Christ. I would review the lives of Job and Paul with them. I would say that even though things often do go well for us when we "do everything right," this blessing is not a guarantee. Therefore, we need to continue to seek God for *who* He is and not act as mercenary worshippers seeking only *what* we can get from Him. I'd also look at passages like Psalm 73 (especially verses 16–17 and 25–28) and Revelation 2:8–11.

Questions About the Christian Life/Witness

If sexuality is moral and not political, how can Christians serve as the light of Christ in a world of utter darkness and depravity?

I will say two things here. First, yes, sexuality is moral and therefore individual and personal. Second, politics is applied theology. Government, in all its forms, seeks to promote what it believes is good, right, and true while opposing that with which it disagrees. The problem lies in situations where what the Christian believes is good, right, and true is not shared by the government. Historically, Christians in the West have been able to assume their values were generally shared by their governments. Unfortunately, this is no longer the case; then again, it has never been the case in places like China, Iran, or North Korea. Christians there have never assumed they would have alignment with the values of their government.

So how should Christians in the West respond, especially those who live in representative democracies? I believe the answer lies in three actions: First, live out your life in such a way that you display words and deeds that are good, right, and true. Let your witness provoke others to want what you have. Second, pray for others. Remember, this is primarily a spiritual war. Ask God to keep the forces of darkness at bay, take back spiritual territory, and turn people's hearts toward Him. Third, participate in government when and where you can. Support candidates who share your views, consider running for office yourself, and talk with people about why they should care about these things. Tom Holland, a British historian, has written and spoken extensively about how a distinctly Christian sexual ethic was a compelling witness for the early church. During that time, most of the sexual depravity we see today was considered commonplace. Yet early Christians lived such different lives that it caught the attention of friends and neighbors who were compelled by this behavior long before the government began to reflect Christian values.[2]

What should the church do to curb the sexual assault on schoolchildren through the transgender movement in our schools? If it's strictly a political issue, we could stay out of the debate for unity's sake, but if it's a moral issue, is it incumbent upon the church to take a stand?

Christians are to be ambassadors for the Kingdom of God. Therefore, we should share the position of our King on this issue: Transgender ideology harms children. However, we need to be prepared for the possibility that our stance will be rejected, just as it often is regarding other areas of sexuality and issues like abortion. Ultimately, what we desire is for such things

---

2. Tom Holland, *Dominion: How the Christian Revolution Remade the World* (Basic Books, 2019). See especially pages 95–98, where Holland discusses how early Christian sexual ethics contrasted sharply with Roman norms by emphasizing chastity, monogamy, and the dignity of all people, including women and slaves.

to become unthinkable rather than merely illegal, but that will not occur until hearts turn to Christ. So, much like the answer to the previous question, we need to live as Christ's witnesses (Acts 1:8), pray for victory in the spiritual aspects of this war, and, when possible, engage in the political process and in conversations with others in efforts to win them to the position of our King.

How can we pray about these issues? How do we prepare to confront those we love?

There are many ways to pray about these issues, but I recommend we not overlook the simplest—to pray the Lord's Prayer: "Our Father in heaven, hallowed be Your name. Your kingdom come. Your will be done on earth as it is in heaven" (Matthew 6:9–10). There's a lot of richness there to be chewed on. Consider how life would change if people hallowed God's name and did His will more often. You can get specific in your prayers, praying for certain people and certain aspects of these issues, but there's also a lot to be gained by praying as Jesus taught us to pray.

When preparing to approach someone on these topics, I like to say, "Pray *for* them more than you talk *to* them." We want heart change more than behavior change, and I believe God has the ability to speak to someone directly in a way that produces deep change and true repentance without us ever opening our mouths. Now, engaging in conversation will need to happen sometimes, but the discussion will go much better if God has also opened their ears to hear and their heart to receive, so pray for that to happen.

Appendix A: Common Questions and Answers

Why do I have to accept what someone else thinks about Scripture when it contradicts what I think? Look at all the Christian denominations and independent churches that don't agree on everything. How can I know who's right?

This is a great question! First, you don't *have* to accept someone else's interpretation of Scripture just because they claim authority. The Bible, not human opinion, is our ultimate standard (2 Timothy 3:16–17). But you're right. Different churches and denominations land on different conclusions. So what should we do?

- **Start with Scripture Itself:** The Bible is God's inspired Word, and it is trustworthy. When interpretations differ, go back to the text. Study the passage in its context—historically, culturally, and grammatically. What's the author's intent? How does it fit with the broader message of Scripture? Tools like concordances, reputable commentaries, or even a good study Bible can help clarify, but always test them against the text itself.

- **Pray for Wisdom:** The Holy Spirit guides believers into truth (John 16:13). Ask God for discernment as you study. He's not going to leave you hanging if you're genuinely seeking Him.

- **Test Interpretations Against Core Truths:** While denominations disagree on secondary issues like baptism, church government, or the end times, the core doctrines of Christianity—salvation by grace through faith, the deity of Christ, the Resurrection—

are nonnegotiable truths shared across Orthodox churches (John 14:6–11; 1 Corinthians 15:3–4). If an interpretation contradicts these essentials, it's likely off base.

- **Consider the Weight of History:** The church has been studying Scripture for two thousand years. Creeds like the Nicene or Apostles' Creed and the writings of early church fathers can provide guardrails (though even these brothers were not infallible!). If your interpretation is brand-new or contradicts what the church has historically affirmed, that's a red flag.

- **Engage in Christian Community:** God gave us the church for a reason (Hebrews 10:24–25). Discuss your questions with trusted, biblically grounded believers or elders. They're not infallible, but they can offer perspective. Iron sharpens iron (Proverbs 27:17), and theology is best understood in community (Ephesians 4:11–16).

- **Accept That True Christ Followers Sometimes Disagree:** Some issues—like the exact timing of Christ's return—are less clear, and godly people can differ in their beliefs. Hold your views with humility, knowing that we all "see in a mirror, dimly" (1 Corinthians 13:12).

- **Focus on What's Clear:** Scripture's main message is unmistakable: God loves you, Christ died for your sins, and you're called to repent and follow Him (John 3:16; Acts 2:38). Don't get so lost in disputes that you miss the forest for the trees.

Appendix A: Common Questions and Answers

No denomination or pastor has a monopoly on truth. Test everything against God's Word (1 Thessalonians 5:21). If you're diligent, humble, and open to the Spirit's leading, you'll grow in confidence about what's true, even amid differing beliefs.

Appendix B: Recommended Resources

Making recommendations is always a tricky thing. This is not meant to be a complete endorsement of every paragraph or sentence written by the authors, but the following resources have proven to be generally helpful and insightful.

General Reference

Andreas J. Köstenberger and David W. Jones, *God, Marriage, and Family: Rebuilding the Biblical Foundation*, 2nd ed. **(Crossway, 2010).** This comprehensive volume offers a thorough biblical theology of marriage, family, sexuality, and gender roles. It's academically and spiritually solid, making it valuable for pastors, counselors, and serious students who want a clear understanding of God's design for these foundational areas of life.

Tony Reinke, *Ask Pastor John: 750 Bible Answers to Life's Most Important Questions* **(Crossway, 2024).** This resource is a collection of responses from the *Ask Pastor*

John podcast that cover a wide range of topics, including sexuality, marriage, suffering, and Christian living. John Piper's answers are edited for clarity and organized topically, making subjects easy to find. Answers range from a paragraph to a few pages and are deeply rooted in Scripture.

Our Current Cultural Moment

Carl R. Trueman, *Strange New World: How Thinkers and Activists Redefined Identity and Sparked the Sexual Revolution* **(Crossway, 2022).** Carl Trueman details the evolution of ideas that brought us to this current cultural moment, addressing the questions "Who taught what and what influence did it have?" This is an excellent resource for those who ask, "How did all of this happen?"

Sexual Addiction and Abuse

David Powlison, *Making All Things New: Restoring Joy to the Sexually Broken* **(Crossway, 2017).** This short and deeply pastoral book offers hope and healing to those struggling with sexual sin or brokenness. David Powlison addresses the heart-level issues behind sexual struggles, grounding his counsel in Scripture and the grace of Christ. It's an especially helpful resource for those seeking both personal renewal and practical help for discipling others.

Appendix B: Recommended Resources

Pornography

Heath Lambert, *Finally Free: Fighting for Purity with the Power of Grace* **(Zondervan, 2013).** This book provides a clear, gospel-centered approach to overcoming pornography. Heath Lambert emphasizes grace-driven transformation over behavior modification while offering concrete strategies for accountability and change.

Ray Ortlund, *The Death of Porn: Men of Integrity Building a World of Nobility* **(Crossway, 2021).** Written as a series of letters from a spiritual father to a younger man, this book challenges the cultural norm of porn use and calls men to live with dignity, purity, and Kingdom-minded purpose.

Tim Challies, *Sexual Detox: A Guide for Guys Who Are Sick of Porn* **(Cruciform Press, 2010).** Tim Challies speaks directly and candidly to men battling pornography, offering both theological clarity and practical advice. This is a brief but potent resource that helps readers understand the damage of porn, renew their minds with truth, and pursue lasting purity.

Technology Use and Its Impact on Our Behaviors

Samuel D. James, *Digital Liturgies: Rediscovering Christian Wisdom in an Online Age* **(Crossway, 2023).** Samuel James explores how the internet's immersive nature shapes our thoughts and behaviors through five "digital liturgies" — authenticity, outrage, shame, consumption, and meaninglessness. James offers valuable insights and practical guidance for Christians seeking to use technology with wisdom. Chapter 7, "Naked in the Dark," is especially helpful regarding pornography.

Same-Sex Attraction and Homosexuality

Kevin DeYoung, *What Does the Bible Really Teach About Homosexuality?* **(Crossway, 2015).** This concise book (about 150 pages) addresses a new question or issue in each chapter, making it easy to find a quick response to your specific inquiry. Kevin DeYoung also tackles each of the so-called "clobber verses" in the Bible that address homosexuality, providing a clear, faithful exegesis of each text.

Out of Egypt Ministries: This ministry, led by Patti Height, offers several resources on its website for those working through various forms of same-sex attraction and sexual struggle (outofegyptministries.org).

Rebecca McLaughlin, *Confronting Christianity: 12 Hard Questions for the World's Largest Religion* **(Crossway, 2019).** This work, by Rebecca McLaughlin (who holds a PhD in English literature from the University of Cambridge and a theology degree from Oak Hill College in London), tackles some of the world's toughest objections to Christianity, including questions about sex, gender, and Christianity's exclusivity as the one true faith. McLaughlin shares her own experience with same-sex attraction and writes with clarity and compassion. This is an excellent resource for skeptics, seekers, and believers alike.

Appendix B: Recommended Resources

Rosaria Champagne Butterfield, *The Secret Thoughts of an Unlikely Convert: An English Professor's Journey into Christian Faith* **(Crown & Covenant Publications, 2012).** As the title of this book indicates, author Rosaria Butterfield shares how she came to the Christian faith, detailing her journey from being a lesbian professor at a progressive university to becoming a pastor's wife.

Healthy Marriage

Timothy Keller and Kathy Keller, *The Meaning of Marriage: Facing the Complexities of Commitment with the Wisdom of God* **(Dutton, 2011).** This foundational book on Christian marriage emphasizes the relationship as a covenantal union that reflects Christ's love for the church, prioritizing mutual sacrifice and spiritual companionship over romantic idealism. Timothy and Kathy Keller draw from their forty-five years of marriage and use insights from Ephesians 5 to provide practical guidance for both singles and couples.

About the Author

Jeff Schlenz is the pastor of The City Gates Church in Fairfax, Virginia. He has dedicated more than twenty years to pastoral ministry, teaching, and counseling people to embrace the blessings that come from submitting to God's authority in every aspect of life. Jeff has served as an assistant pastor, a missions pastor, a military chaplain (colonel, US Air Force), and a senior pastor. He holds a master of arts in intercultural studies (missions), a master of divinity, and a doctor of ministry from Liberty Theological Seminary in Lynchburg, Virginia. Along with his wife, Madeleine, he has published numerous Turn Aside Bible studies designed to encourage people to engage with Scripture personally. Jeff and Madeleine have three children and live in the suburbs of Washington, DC.

www.ingramcontent.com/pod-product-compliance
Lightning Source LLC
Chambersburg PA
CBHW020541030426
42337CB00013B/937